AM I MY BROTHER'S KEEPER?

Medical Ethics series

David H. Smith and Robert M. Veatch, Editors

AM I MY BROTHER'S KEEPER?

THE ETHICAL FRONTIERS OF BIOMEDICINE

Arthur L. Caplan

INDIANA UNIVERSITY PRESS   BLOOMINGTON AND INDIANAPOLIS

THE PAPER USED IN THIS PUBLICATION MEETS THE MINI-
MUM REQUIREMENTS OF AMERICAN NATIONAL STANDARD FOR
INFORMATION SCIENCES—PERMANENCE OF PAPER FOR
PRINTED LIBRARY MATERIALS, ANSI Z39.48-1984.

MANUFACTURED IN THE UNITED STATES OF AMERICA

LIBRARY OF CONGRESS CATALOGING-IN-PUBLICATION DATA

Caplan, Arthur L.
AM I MY BROTHER'S KEEPER? : THE ETHICAL FRONTIERS
OF BIOMEDICINE / ARTHUR L. CAPLAN.
P.   CM. — (MEDICAL ETHICS SERIES)
INCLUDES BIBLIOGRAPHICAL REFERENCES AND INDEX.
ISBN 0-253-33358-X (CLOTH : ALK. PAPER)
1. MEDICAL ETHICS. I. TITLE. II. SERIES.
R724.C337 1997
174'.2—DC21   97-19268

3 4 5 02 01 00 99

CONTENTS

PREFACE

No one writes a book alone. Spouses and children have to put up with the time lost to the task. The advice of former teachers and mentors rings in the writer's head. The whispers of present and former colleagues and students create a background hum that makes it very difficult to identify whose ideas are really present on any given page. And the kindness of those willing to put up with silly questions or desperate requests for support infuses nearly every page.

I am especially grateful to my son, Zachary, and my wife, Jane, who show little tolerance for my obsession about my work and force me to stay engaged with what is truly important in life. And I would like to thank my colleagues at the University of Pennsylvania, who have created a wonderful climate for thinking about the hard issues that advances in biomedicine raise.

INTRODUCTION

When I was a boy a place called Boys Town used to advertise itself on television, billboards, and stickers and in magazines with a picture accompanied by a slogan. Most people who have heard of this institution know about it from a movie by the same name that starred Spencer Tracy. But Boys Town was not just the stuff of cinematic fantasy. It was and remains a home in Nebraska for kids from troubled families. Some kids found a home there because they were orphans. Others had parents who left them or from whom they had become estranged. I had watched Spencer Tracy play the role of the kindly but tough Boys Town priest, Father Flanagan, in the movie. But it was the ads that made a real impression on me.

The ads used an instantly recognizable picture and a slogan. The picture was of a boy in his teens carrying an even younger boy piggyback. The slogan was "He ain't heavy, he's my brother." The point of the advertisement was to show both that a brother would not find it burdensome to carry a sibling in need on his back and to subtly suggest that Boys Town did not find it burdensome to try to help kids with all sorts of problems make it in the world.

The notion that we view one another as brothers and consequently pitch in to help one another make it through this world strikes a lot of people today as, at best, corny and, at worst, just plain stupid. When I show the old Boys Town ad to my students, most merely smile and shake their heads, disbelieving that anyone they know could ever have taken the sentiment and sentimentality in the ad seriously.

Why does the notion of helping others leave so many of us cold? The question is not merely one of historical or cultural interest. A good many of the moral problems that Americans find themselves confronting in their health care system stem from their unwillingness to carry anyone else on their back, even briefly and even when it is a family member. Our society has grown so enamored of personal freedom and self-determination that any act of charity, kindness, or beneficence seems extraordinary. Helping another is the kind of act that moralists refer to as supererogatory—going beyond the call of duty or obligation. Giving money to charity, spending an afternoon delivering meals to the poor, or a company's sharing its earnings with its employees seems so out of character, so morally unexpected, that it becomes the stuff of high praise and sometimes even media celebration. This is so even when, as in the case of the boy carrying his brother on his back in the old Boys Town ads, the act of generosity is not especially onerous and is one which any decent person ought to undertake willingly and eagerly.

Bioethics is no less afflicted with egoism than any other arena of life in the United States. There is much talk of rights and hardly any of duties. Every nuance of freedom and personal self-determination receives close scrutiny in doctor-patient relations but precious little attention is paid to what bonds built on trust, friendship, and caring would impose on those engaged in an attempt to heal or palliate. Everyone wants to expound on who really deserves a heart or liver transplant, but few seem to have the stomach for a discussion of why it is that thousands of Americans are never even considered for a transplant because of their age, lack of health insurance, or lack of access to decent primary care.

True, there is much talk of community and of civil discourse today in many seminar rooms, editorial offices, and think tanks. But all too often these discussions are about how a people immersed in autonomy can manage to talk with and to one another without literally killing each other. Serious calls for beneficence, for acting compassionately or in a kind manner to one another, or for the government to do its duty to those in need are not much in evidence. The expectation that anyone would go out of his or her way to do good for others, much less that kindness and compassion would be expected, does not exist. About the best the United States society can do, immersed as it is in a sea of self-determination, is to post an occasional unintentionally ironic bumper sticker urging random acts of kindness. How did we get to such a parlous state of moral affairs, one with such nasty consequences for each other and for those facing ethical issues in health care?

Americans who had clung together through the Great Depression and two long world wars, who saw themselves in the 1950s and early 1960s as a nation dutybound to help those less fortunate both in this country and abroad could look at that ad for Boys Town and believe in its moral message. And they expected their kids to believe that message, too. Today's Americans, who have watched their government dissemble and lie, who have seen authorities and agencies engage in coverups and conspiracies from Watergate to Iran-Contra to the presence of chemical weapons in the Gulf War, whose leaders seem constantly mired in moral quagmires and personal scandal, who have endured decades of being feared and hated by many of the world's people, some of whom seemed intent on nothing less than their annihilation, who find themselves awash in a sea of violence and racial strife both in real life and in their media and entertainment, have grown wary, skeptical, and cynical. They do not trust their neighbors, much less foreigners. They are more likely to march for animal rights than human rights. A smirk is the most an ad like the one for Boys Town can be expected to produce. "I'll get mine" and "Look out for number one" are the slogans most likely to resonate in the contemporary American ear as an ethos to live by. Today's Boys Town ad, to be realistic, would need to have an adolescent lugging a boy on his back with the slogan "He is pretty heavy, but I got paid twenty bucks to carry him so I will for a while."

Moral cynicism is rife in our classrooms and in our public discourse. Pessimism is not far behind. Few Americans really believe that people when given a choice will do the ethical thing. Disregard what social scientists say. Ask your relatives at your next family gathering whether they think people try to do the right thing or will do the right thing if they think it is possible to get away with being immoral, and you will see what I mean. There is pessimism about whether it is even possible to talk about ethical issues in a pluralistic society such as the one in the United States. In a society of many religions, races, and creeds, relativism is more than a question of passing theoretical interest. For many Americans it is hard to distinguish between respect for cultural and religious differences and simply accepting that different people have different values and that is that.

In the area I know best, the ethics of health care, cynicism and pessimism abound. When I explain to people that I am interested in ethical issues in health care, many simply smile, as if I had declared myself to be mildly retarded. Others want to know how it is possible to examine ethical issues if there is no agreement on a religious foundation for moral values. Still others wonder why I would want to serve as an apologist for the powerful forces of medicine, the pharmaceutical industry, the nursing home industry, malpractice lawyers, unions, and managed care companies. And members of the media find themselves unable to imagine a world in which ethics is not lagging so far behind where technology and science are headed that the only function an ethicist can play is to mop up with woe and remorse after the biomedical disaster, damage, or debacle is over.

But the cynicism and pessimism about the power of ethics in society generally and in medicine in particular is misplaced. It is simply not true that it is impossible to reach moral consensus without a common starting point or foundational theory. Anyone who doubts this contention need only look at the moral revolution that has swept through medicine with respect to truth telling, disclosure, consent, and the treatment of subjects in research in the past half-century. Agreement on intermediate values, such as the importance of autonomy and the need to respect individual dignity, has led to moral consensus about what health care providers should do and what patients can reasonably expect from their doctors, nurses, and other providers.

The moral problems that seem endemic to modern medicine are not a function of the failure to find the right fundamental moral theory. Nor are they the product of biomedicine's running too far ahead of morality. Rather, moral disquiet and cynicism, at least as they extend into the realm of health care, are very much a function of social, economic, and cultural change in modern society.

To put the diagnosis simply, we are not certain whether we can trust one another any longer. It is not that we cannot communicate about our value differences. Cultural diversity does not lead, as many would argue, to incommensurability—the inability to communicate. People understand very well what is meant when talking about rationing health care or the moral acceptability of abortion or forced sterilization. Communication across the cultural and religious divide is not the problem. Distrust of who is on the other side of the divide is.

Levels of distrust run deep in the modern hospital, clinic, nursing home, and waiting room. When those involved in health care relationships are strangers, trust is not strong. When those involved in health care come from different economic and social backgrounds, trust has a hard time flourishing. And when the goal of health policy emphasizes more and more the need to constrain resources rather than patient self-interest, the prospects for trust are threatened.

The primary reason bioethics seems so hard and to some simply impossible is that we have lost our faith in our ability to see others as our brothers. Instead we view our doctors as our enemies, our insurers as our adversaries, those who make our drugs and devices as plotting to rip us off, and each other when seriously ill as at best burdens who must be carried rather than as fragile members of a community who need our help much as we will someday need theirs.

one

And Baby Makes—Moral Muddles

WHAT LAWS GOVERN THE CREATION of babies? For Americans making children the old-fashioned way, through sexual reproduction, surprisingly few. It is against the law to force someone to have sexual relations, in nearly every state it is illegal to pay for sex in order to reproduce, and there are various state laws governing the age at which someone may consent to sex. Few other legal constraints exist. The situation is not much different when medical technology is used to make a baby. But it is not at all clear that the minimal regulation that suffices in the bedroom is sufficient for the clinic laboratory.

There is a widespread belief that the techniques of assisted reproduction such as artificial insemination by donor and in vitro fertilization are among the most tightly regulated, closely monitored areas in all of health care. Many argue that the legal climate governing the making of babies using artificial means is, if anything, too restrictive (Robertson, 1994, 1995; Christensen, Kelleher, Nicolosi, and Parrish, 1995; King, 1995; Wozencraft, 1996). Defenders of the status quo contend that with the exception of the occasional oddball patient, rogue practitioner or outlaw clinic, there is no reason for concern about the field of artificial reproduction. Surely the government has no business trying to regulate who it is that can use or provide biomedical technology to make a child. Business ethics, a combination of professional self-restraint and consumer savvy, is sufficient to keep the making of babies on an even moral keel.

Americans are so enamored of self-determination that it is difficult to make a case in favor of more societal intervention and oversight and less individual choice. There are, however, many reasons to think that unfettered self-determination is not enough to govern the lucrative business of making babies. Part of the reason why autonomy seems sufficient as a moral foundation for the new reproductive technologies is a reflection of the narrow moral focus that accompanied their birth.

The first baby created using in vitro fertilization, the mixing of sperm and egg outside the human body in a plastic dish, was Louise Brown. She was born in England in 1978. Much moral controversy preceded her birth.

The main moral problem with making babies outside the human body was safety. Would fertilization in a glass dish result in a healthy child? Before the birth of Louise Brown, no human being had ever originated outside the environment of a womb. There was real concern about whether this mode of origin was safe. While other issues were raised as to the unnaturalness of conception outside the womb, the moral worry that had real clout was the safety of the procedure. It seemed to many unethical to risk deformity or death using a new procedure on a child who could not consent to these risks (Caplan, 1992a).

The issue was solved when a pair of British scientists, with little fanfare and no societal approbation, went ahead and performed the experiment. The result, which appeared nine months later, was a quite healthy Louise Brown. The critics of artificial conception outside the human body either fell silent or were no longer heard. Safety was no longer an issue.

Since that time, the field of assisted reproduction has evolved with token external regulation and, in the United States, an ostrichlike posture on the part of legislators in the face of growing societal unease about the intersection of biomedical technology and the making of babies. If safety was the compelling source of moral worry about making babies in "test tubes," then the safety issue was resolved by the production in this way of thousands of healthy babies. Serious moral debate about the artificial creation of children subsequently moved from the realm of public policy to the odd seminar or two at a university or think tank.

In recent years there has been a disturbingly lengthy parade of crises, scandals, and abuses involving vulnerable persons who have sought medical help in having a child (Mydans, 1995). The level of misconduct and uncertainty may be sufficient to send the question of what two

Our collective obsession with autonomy has blinded us to the need to rely upon one another at moments of weakness, illness, and death. Our policies and laws are so consumed with individual rights that the moral framework upon which we need to rely when autonomy and self-determination are impaired or absent—virtues, beneficence, trust—are given short shrift.

The essays in this book time and time again point toward trust as a vital necessity for Americans faced with the daunting task of navigating our way around the bedside and the boardroom, through situations that determine how we live and how we die. Deciding to help one another carry the inevitable and unavoidable burdens of illness, disability, and dying is not only possible and prudent; it is the right and minimally decent thing to do.

PART ONE

RESEARCH, EXPERIMENTATION, AND INNOVATION

decades of unfettered, free-market entrepreneurism have done to the field of reproductive technology back up to the front burner of public policy. If more is not done to monitor and control how the technology is used, then not only will people continue to be harmed and mistreated in the course of seeking assistance in having a child, but there may well be a societal backlash against the continued application of technology and scientific knowledge to the creation of human life. That would be unfortunate.

Persons who are infertile, those who are fertile but whose lives are at risk should they become pregnant, and those who might transmit grave genetic disorders to their children have benefited greatly from reproductive technologies such as in vitro fertilization. Ask any parents of a child conceived by technological means if they are grateful to the doctors and techniques that allowed the miracle to happen and you had better be prepared to listen for a long time. What is not so obvious is whether the technology can be kept on a moral leash of sufficient strength to ensure that the rights, dignity, and interests of those who use it or who are created from it are adequately protected.

The argument for the preservation of the status quo with respect to assisted reproduction rests on the assumption that reproduction is and must remain an activity where individual choice is supreme (Robertson, 1994, 1995; Baker, 1995; Walsh, 1994). If people have a fundamental right, both moral and legal, to privacy and freedom when it comes to reproduction, then there is no other value that can justify intervening with whatever it is they decide to do. Once individual choice is posited as the sole value that ought to guide all reproduction, natural or artificially mediated, it is only a small step to the argument that an unregulated free market is the best vehicle for delivering assisted reproductive services (Boone, 1992; Wozencraft, 1996), since markets are arguably the most effective means for responding to individual choice.

There is no point in discussing what norms ought to govern assisted reproduction unless a case can be made for more oversight and accountability in the face of this powerful commitment to personal freedom and self-determination. A case can be made. The notion that self-determination is all that matters when artificial reproductive technologies are used to make babies is simply wrong. And the notion that with a few exceptions there are no problems worthy of societal concern in the domain of reproductive technology also is wrong.

Two conceptual problems surround the argument that individual choice is enough in making babies. The first is the equation of the freedom to be free from interference in making a choice with the idea that freedom entails the ability to have any and all assistance required to fulfill that choice. The freedom requisite for personal self-determination, freedom from interference, is not the same as the freedom to act on any preference or choice, to be entitled to any and all things which might be desired.

Those who argue that no one should interfere in deeply personal matters of reproductive choice are partially correct. Any interference by the government or third parties in reproductive decisions requires a powerful moral justification, since the moral presumption is that individuals should be free to decide how many children they want and when they want them without outside interference. This sort of procreative freedom, what is sometimes termed negative freedom, is widely recognized in numerous international codes of human rights and many United States laws and court decisions (Overall, 1987).

There is no basis to the claim that individuals have a positive right to the means necessary to implement their choices (Overall, 1987). If I wish to reproduce, the state is not obliged to supply me with a willing partner or a hired surrogate. There is no entitlement to the means necessary to have a child, natural or technological, even though I am free to reproduce if I wish to do so. Moreover, the absence of any entitlement means that the state and third parties are not prohibited from placing certain conditions or requirements on those who wish to use or require artificial means in order to reproduce.

Choice, in order to have value, must be real. If persons are operating with only the illusion of choice, if some choices lead to practices that undermine the possibility of real choice, then choice is an empty value (Raymond, 1993). If those who seek reproductive services are not adequately informed of their options, risks, and benefits, they do not have real freedom and cannot make real choices. If, for example, choices are made about how many embryos to create, how many to implant, and how to track and store frozen gametes, reproductive materials, and embryos without discussion with the parties supplying them and if those providing reproductive services do not provide accurate and timely information about the risks of fertility-enhancing drugs, success rates using different techniques, and costs, then choice is illusory, especially in an area as sensitive and as defining of personal self-image as reproduction (Raymond, 1993).

The strongest reason for infringing on personal self-determination with respect to reproduction is that others may be adversely affected by the choices individuals make. Others' interests need to be taken into account in deciding how far self-determination ought go in creating new lives.

It makes sense to put limits on personal choice with respect to assisted reproduction, even though similar restrictions do not exist for sexual reproduction, because of the unique kinds of harms that may and have befallen a significant number of those who have used reproductive technologies. Some people have been unknowingly put at risk by receiving high doses of fertility drugs. Others have been harmed because their wishes have not been followed with respect to the handling of their embryos or eggs. Some have been wronged because providers have not given them accurate information or a full range of options for dealing with their infertility. Some have been harmed by not being made fully aware of the potential financial costs associated with multiple births and the dangers of disability associated with premature birth and multiple pregnancy for both baby and mother (Collins, 1994). Choice is often less than it seems in assisted reproduction. Too often choice and informed consent are used as shields to defend the interests of provider and insurer rather than of those seeking reproduction assistance and their offspring.

So the right to reproduce is not a reason why values other than self-determination should not be brought to bear on the matter of how babies are made. The proliferation of scandals and problems in the field of reproductive technology shows that it is essential to consider values other than self-determination if the interests of children and their parents are to be protected.

The field of technologically assisted reproduction has been beset in recent years by a series of flagrant and egregious moral violations (Caplan, 1995a; Freyer, 1995; Mydans, 1995). In many cases the parties who were harmed could not have protected themselves against the mistakes, deception, or fraud involved. These scandals are troubling in terms of harms done to patients seeking treatment for reproductive problems and to the children created in the course of these events. The level of scandal in recent years is such as to make the case for the adequacy of an unregulated, unaccountable free market in reproductive services entirely implausible.

Assisted reproduction, unlike sexual reproduction, is a social enterprise. It requires the involvement of many third parties as well as significant amounts of social resources. In ordinary circumstances, individuals do not need society's help to make babies. In extraordinary circumstances, they can only do so with that help. What level of help society is willing to tolerate, provide, or pay for moves assisted reproduction beyond the boundaries of personal choice and individual liberty. Whether the marketplace has sufficed as a moral rudder in the past (Robertson, 1994) is debatable. An unregulated market will not prove adequate for keeping artificial reproduction on a moral course in the future.

Making Babies without Permission—The UC-Irvine Scandal

In the United States, ethical or legal oversight is often the response to scandal. A whopper of a scandal is sometimes needed to attract sufficient public attention to change public policy. The field of assisted reproduction has had such a scandal. The mess at the University of California at Irvine's Center for Reproductive Health is of sufficient dimension and scope to impugn the adequacy of the current ethical, regulatory, legal, and legislative state of affairs with respect to the creation of babies by technological means (Caplan, 1995c; Christensen, Kelleher, Nicolosi, and Parrish, 1995; Mydans, 1995; Robertson, 1995).

The scandal became public as a result of the courageous actions of a small number of administrators and technicians who worked at the UC-Irvine infertility clinic. They felt morally obligated to raise concerns about the conduct of the doctors running the clinic. Their complaints to state and federal officials revealed misconduct of staggering proportions.

Dr. Ricardo Asch was the director of the center. His record as a pioneer in the field of reproductive technology, both as a clinician and as a researcher, was impressive. He was a leader in the field right up to 1995, when he left the United States as the scandal in his program became public.

Dr. Asch apparently obtained embryos from patients who were trying to conceive and used them to create children for other patients who had sought his care. As many as one hundred women may have had their eggs or embryos used without their explicit consent. No one obtained the explicit permission of the recipients of these stolen embryos. A number of infertility centers, some outside California, unknowingly used stolen embryos from the Asch clinic. Not all embryos were used to make babies. Some were shipped outside the state for research purposes.

When concerns about the handling of embryos in Asch's program first began to surface, the Irvine administrators launched an internal investigation. But it moved slowly and seemed devoted primarily to not causing problems for the university. Frustrated by the tortoiselike pace of the Irvine inquiry and fearing that nothing would be done to punish the doctors involved, a whistle-blower from the Irvine clinic contacted me early in the fall of 1994. I arranged a meeting at a Philadelphia hotel with a number of federal officials I trusted.

Everyone in the hotel room was flabbergasted by the story the whistle-blower told. Systematic wrongdoing had taken place over a considerable period. I offered a number of suggestions as to what course the whistle-blower might want to pursue. Some of them were pursued. A few months later, subpoenas began to fly around California, and the state's media, especially the *Orange County Register*, which eventually won a Pulitzer Prize for its coverage, began to follow the scandal closely.

If no one had gone outside the institution to attract attention to the theft at UC-Irvine, if the whistle-blowers had remained silent when offered generous cash settlements, the scandal probably would not have become public and the physicians at the clinic would still be practicing there. The sole reason why the events at Irvine became known was that administrators and technicians put their careers on the line by raising questions about what was taking place at this internationally renowned program.

There is a peculiar aspect to the Irvine scandal. In sum, what was happening is that the doctors were making babies. It is odd to complain about the creation of life. Embryos stored in liquid nitrogen will not become people. Couples who cannot create embryos can, if stored embryos are used, have children that are very much wanted. Until whistles were blown, presumably the babies that were made using spare embryos were happy, and so were their parents. Where is the moral problem?

Using an artificially created frozen embryo to make a baby is a wonder of modern medicine. Stealing one to do so is not.

The theft of embryos to create children for others constitutes a terrible betrayal of trust. Creating a new life without permission of the person whose gametes are used is a violation of the most intimate areas of privacy, dignity, and self-determination. Whether through outright theft or simply error, the creation of a child without the consent of those whose gametes are used to do so is a fundamental violation of human dignity (Elliot and Endt, 1995). As the identity of donors and recipients in the stolen embryo scandal at UC-Irvine are traced, highly emotional battles will ensue between the gamete donors and those who have been rearing the children produced from the gametes unaware that the embryos which provided them with their child were stolen.

Making babies without consent was the most serious but apparently not the only misconduct in the program. Fiscal hanky-panky concerning overcharging for patient services and drugs, as well as the use of cheap imported fertility drugs never approved by the Food and Drug Administration, was among the crimes that may have occurred at the Irvine clinic.

The scandal is symptomatic of a much deeper problem that has haunted the field of assisted reproduction since its inception. While the goal of assisting infertile men and women in having babies is worthy, the motives of some of those providing reproductive services are not. Money and even greed are too often in evidence where the creation of children is concerned.

Infertility treatment is big business in the United States (Freudenheim, 1996). Patients pay from $6,000 to $12,000 for a single attempt at in vitro fertilization. Four, five, or more attempts are not uncommon. Asch and his associates at UC-Irvine reported earnings of $4.5 million over the last three years of their practice in California. Their ability to charge high prices and make big profits was an important reason why UC-Irvine aggressively recruited Asch and his group to come out from Texas.

Money is also the reason why there are so many infertility clinics in the United States today. Money is the reason why some clinics have turned to offering their patients rebates and money-back guarantees as a way to ensure their patient flow in the face of high fees and an unwillingness on the part of many public and private insurers to pay them. And money is the reason why the field of infertility treatment and reproductive technology continues to evolve in the United States with no oversight, minimal regulation, and no moral guideposts.

A Year's Worth of Problems

Fifteen years ago, fewer than five programs were offering test-tube baby technology in the United States. Today there are hundreds. The same story can be told for sperm banks and egg-donor and surrogacy programs. There are too many infertility programs relative to the need and demand for services. Some centers are scandalously unproficient at treating infertility. Quality control, as the Irvine scandal clearly shows, is not up to par. The procedures used to keep track of embryos and other reproductive materials are so poor that it is not possible to weed out inept or unethical practitioners and facilities. And, sadly, the events surrounding the conduct of Dr. Asch at a premier infertility program with the reputation and standing that UC-Irvine's had cannot be dismissed as nothing more than an aberration or as the actions of a single bad apple.

Consider only the issue of keeping track of embryos. Problems in this area were not confined to Irvine in 1995.

On July 26, 1995, David and Carol Frisina filed suit in Superior Court in Providence, Rhode Island, charging that the infertility program at Rhode Island's Women & Infants Hospital could not account for six of their embryos. This suit was followed by another one against the same institution: Vicki and Robert Lamontagne asserted that the hospital was unable to locate three of their embryos (Freyer, 1995). Two other couples also came forward publicly to complain about the mishandling of embryos at the same institution.

While the loss of the embryos may have been unavoidable, the failure to inform the couples in a timely manner that their embryos no longer existed was not. There is no established and universal procedure in the United States for assuring couples that embryos they have stored remain stored or that they have been used in ways that conform with their makers' wishes.

Impunity in mishandling embryos and a lack of quality control are hardly the only problems facing those who provide or use infertility services. Other scandals have ripped through the field of reproductive technology. A review of some of the most notorious for a single year provides a litany of moral lapses and failures sufficient in number and magnitude to give pause to even the staunchest defenders of free choice and free markets as the only values that ought to guide the making of babies.

In the first week of December 1995, the Genetics and IVF Institute in Fairfax, Virginia, mailed out letters to tens of thousands of physicians in North America who specialize in the treatment of cancer. The letters announced that for a fee of $3,000 to $4,000, doctors at the institute would remove a woman's ovary and store it so that a portion could be returned to her body at a later date (Kolata, 1995). Ovary transplant is of special interest to the tens of thousands of women of childbearing age who undergo chemotherapy and radiation treatment each year. The treatment can destroy their ovaries, leaving them infertile.

The most immediate problem with this form of biological insurance is that there is no evidence that it will work. The first research article on ovarian transplants appeared in a professional journal in 1994. In this study, the technique worked, but the subjects were not women but a small number of sheep (Gosden et al. 1994). No data exists showing that an ovary can be removed, frozen, and stored, then later be put back again so as to function properly in a human female. The procedure is completely experimental, with unknown effects both for the women who might utilize a frozen ovary and for any children who might be made from such tissue. Women desperate to find some way of preserving their fertility thus are being recruited by this Virginia group to spend thousands of dollars on a procedure even though there is not a shred of evidence that it works. Marketing a completely untested procedure as a therapy completely corrodes choice, because it permits a patient to act without full and complete information.

But the problem with efforts at recruiting large numbers of women to store their ovaries does not end with the absence of any hard evidence that the technique works. Putting a transplanted ovary back into a woman who has been cured of cancer might set off a recurrence of her cancer. And there is no way to know whether a baby born from eggs produced by an ovary that has been frozen and thawed will be normal.

Earlier in 1995, on September 12, nine men who stored their sperm with Idant Laboratories, the largest sperm bank in New York State, went to court to prevent anyone from moving their deposits. The State Health Department had closed Idant down after inspectors found hundreds of health and safety violations at the private facility, including a failure to screen sperm donors for infectious diseases. Men had stored sperm at Idant just before undergoing treatments for cancer that left them sterile. The men were concerned that their sperm might be destroyed if moved. No federal or state laws govern the rights of sperm donors in such situations.

On August 7 the same year, James Alan Austin, a single, twenty-six-year-old bank analyst from Hanover Township, Pennsylvania, pled guilty in a northeast Pennsylvania courtroom to killing his son, one-month-old Jonathan Alan Austin. The child had died of a fractured skull and numerous other internal injuries while being treated in the intensive care unit of Children's Hospital of Philadelphia on January 17, 1995. Austin admitted shaking the baby so hard that he damaged the child's brain (Caplan, 1995a).

How did this single man come to have a baby? Austin had paid $30,000 to the Infertility Center of America in Indianapolis to find him a surrogate mother. Clients do not need to appear at the center to undergo screening, and Austin underwent no psychological screening or social work assessment before paying his fee. The mother, Phyllis Huddleston of Lafayette, Indiana, sued Austin and the fertility clinic for damages after the murder of the baby she had sold to him. Whether she has any claim to damages is not clear, since she sold her baby under a surrogacy arrangement and it is not known whether these contracts are valid or not.

There are no federal and practically no state laws restricting who can use infertility services, requiring any sort of psychological testing of the clients of infertility and surrogacy programs, or setting any limits on who can make contracts to buy babies (Covington, 1995). In contrast to adoption procedures, anyone of any age with any type of criminal record or mental illness can seek and hire a surrogate. No federal law governs the practice of commercial surrogacy even though surrogate brokers have long operated across state lines.

In July 1995 a Dutch couple revealed that owing to an error at a fertility clinic, their twin boys had different fathers. One child was white and the other black. Officials at the clinic in Utrecht admitted that the births had probably been the result of reusing an improperly cleaned set of equipment from an earlier in vitro fertilization. The parents insisted that the second biological father be notified, and he was. The parents were furious that no one was punished for the error or that no steps were announced to ensure better quality control at fertility clinics. The parents complained that they had to contend with the assumption of neighbors and friends that the wife had had an extramarital affair. Their black child also faced serious prejudice in Dutch society.

At the beginning of 1995, on January 18, Justice Angelo D. Roncallo of the Supreme Court of New York ruled in a dispute between a Long Island couple, Steven and Maureen Kent Kass, that frozen embryos were solely Maureen's property. Even though the couple had divorced, she wanted to use the embryos to have a baby. The judge's ruling, which was immediately appealed, was completely at odds with a 1992 Tennessee decision, *Davis v. Davis,* that the consent of both parents was necessary before a frozen embryo could be used after a couple divorced. There are no federal or state laws clarifying the legal status of frozen embryos; nor are there any laws to guide courts about what to do with respect to custody should parents divorce, die, or become incapacitated.

Scandal and controversy, as these snapshots of the events of a single year make clear, are not rare in the realm of assisted reproduction. But scandal is incompatible with choice. If persons cannot trust their health care providers, then choice is meaningless. If the incompetent and the malicious can freely avail themselves of infertility services, then choice becomes a vehicle for abuse and harm. And if there are insufficient guidelines to reconcile conflicts when those seeking reproductive assistance make different choices, then fairness, equity, and justice become nothing more than a function of who can back their choices with more resources, better lawyers, and louder press releases.

The list of horrors that a review of a single year's events in the field of assisted reproduction produces is not the end of the story when it comes to examining the adequacy of unfettered free choice in the marketplace as the moral foundation for assisted reproduction. Many other issues and problems are emerging in this field, and they demand more ethical guidance than individual choice can readily provide.

Whether it is a fertile woman who uses drugs to enhance her fertility so that she can have a child with a man who is not her husband, a woman who decides to abort one of the twins she is carrying to lessen the financial burden of parenting, a father who seeks to hire a surrogate to carry one of his deceased twenty-eight-year-old daughter's twelve frozen embryos to term (Craig, 1996), a mother and father who decide to try to freeze the sperm of their unexpectedly deceased teenage son so that their family line can be continued, or a woman who decides to freeze tissues after an abortion in the hope that someday techniques will be found to allow the reanimation of the aborted fetus (Caplan, 1996a), individual choice looks inadequate as a value to ensure that the interests of all parties involved in the creation of children are respected.

The questions raised by advances in reproductive technology are hardly limited to the nonconsensual switching of embryos or the use of unapproved fertility drugs without informed consent on the part of a woman or her partner. Should women in their late fifties and sixties use technology to try to have a child? What sort of counseling if any should an older woman be asked to undergo before she has a baby at sixty or sixty-five? Can a baby develop normally in an older woman's uterus? Should unprecedented pregnancies in older women be viewed as experimental and reviewed by human experimentation committees? Personal choice and individual reproductive freedom provide few answers to these questions.

Is it ethical and should it be legal to pay young women to take fertility drugs so their eggs can be harvested for use by others? Should there not be standardized consent forms and counseling arrangements for young women who may be eager for cash to the point where they do not consider the risks posed to their health by the drugs they must take? How many embryos should be used in each attempt to make a baby? What sort of psychological screening should prospective surrogate mothers receive? What pay if any is appropriate for egg donors or surrogates—whatever the market will bear? Should the citizens of other nations be allowed to come to the United States to find egg and sperm donors when these technologies do not exist or are scorned for religious or cultural reasons in their home countries? Must they agree to disclose the circumstances of their child's creation should the child wish to know or need to know for medical reasons at some future date? Your guess is as good as mine, because none of these questions are covered by law, policy, or regulation.

The case for restraining individual liberty by greater regulatory oversight is especially compelling when one surveys the conceptual bog that is the current state of the law for resolving disputes when choices conflict with respect to reproductive technology. The law has much to say when children are produced by ordinary sexual means, but when conflicts have arisen with respect to potential or actual reproduction accomplished with technological assistance, the law has little to say about how to resolve them. Parties battling over parental rights, access to reproductive services, or custody and control over stored reproductive materials find themselves at the mercy of the discretion of local health care providers, judges, prosecutors, and the media. Choice is not sufficient as an ethos of reproduction if there are no clear rules for adjudicating the consequences of the choices that arise when technological means are used to make babies.

The vacuum that is the law governing assisted reproduction is big enough that judges have issued numerous pleas for legislative guidance as to how the legal system ought to deal with disputes over control, custody, paternity, and ownership in the realm of artificially making babies. The inability of courts to work out satisfactory, much less consistent, resolutions to so many thorny issues—such as determining the custody of embryos when parents divorce, die, or develop dementia; the enforceability of commercial surrogacy contracts; the rights of those involved in paid egg-donor and surrogacy arrangements; and the right of persons to use gametes or embryos long after the sources have died—shows that respect for liberty and choice is not sufficient as a moral foundation for the artificial creation of babies. Worse, assisted reproduction is at risk of having a single court decision bring important research or therapeutic activities to an abrupt halt (Charo, 1995; Annas, Caplan, and Elias, 1996).

Areas abound where technology and new knowledge will greatly expand the opportunity to shape the creation of new lives. Yet little societal discussion has centered on whether these doors ought be opened and, if so, how wide. While choice is important in matters of reproduction, it is not clear that the range and degree of choice afforded by new knowledge and treatments is such that society will want to accord complete freedom to those who make use of assisted reproduction. That is especially so if the children created by assisted reproduction face dangers, risks, and problems that do not ordinarily arise with traditional modes of making babies.

The only ethic that prevails in using technology to make babies is this one: if you have the money, you can find a provider willing to indulge your wishes. Risks, harms, and dangers to you and the resulting child need not be given much weight in an area of medicine where personal choice and the business ethic prevail. Clearly this ethic is inadequate in using new technologies to create new lives.

The numerous incidents I have cited of blatant misconduct, fraud, and immorality, all of which took place in a single year, show that freedom and choice are necessary but not sufficient for using medicine to make babies. The capacity for wrongdoing in the creation of babies, enhanced as it is by the vulnerability of those seeking a child and the pecuniary motives of some offering services, requires that society rely on more than the good graces of ethically minded courageous whistle-blowers and well-intentioned, responsible practitioners.

Can our courts resolve these moral quandaries? Not only are courts unable to reliably detect fraud and misconduct when it does occur in the artificial creation of life; they have no idea what to do with this new technology. Many judges, confronted by the kinds of cases which took place in 1995, know that the adversarial setting of a courtroom is a poor place to resolve matters of parenting, of the creation of life, and of what is in society's best interest in allowing technology to be used to make babies.

Roads with No Maps

As bad as the scandals have been in recent years, reproductive technology continues to develop new ways to make babies. For these new reproductive roads, society has been provided with no maps, few guideposts, and no speed limits. Consider some emerging areas where personal choice provides no guide to the application of reproductive technology.

BECOMING A FATHER AFTER DEATH

Anthony and Maribel Baez were married in June 1992. While visiting relatives for Christmas in the Bronx, New York, two-and-a-half years later, Anthony, a twenty-nine-year-old machine shop operator from Orlando, Florida, was involved in an altercation with police and died on a street corner. In October 1996 the police officers involved were found not guilty of using excessive force. Even after the death of her husband, Maribel Baez apparently still hoped to become pregnant by using sperm that was surgically removed from her dead husband's body.

The ability to make a baby long after a man has died is yet another strange twist resulting from advances in reproductive technology. Some hard questions need to be asked about the morality of taking sperm from the dead.

Whenever a man dies, should sperm retrieval be offered to his loved ones? Many Americans routinely carry organ donor cards. Should these include sections about postmortem donations of sperm? And who should have access to reproductive materials? Is a marriage license enough, or should the stated, written intent on the part of the deceased to someday have children be required? That is the policy which prevails in the United Kingdom, where a young woman, Diane Blood, found herself unable to obtain the sperm of her deceased husband, who had not made a written bequest of it to her.

If reproductive materials are stored, as happened in the Baez case, then how long should they be kept before being either used or destroyed? Will society confer legal recognition and benefits upon children conceived in this manner? And the questions will not stop with the postmortem procurement of sperm. The technology is not yet here for freezing eggs, but women who are deceased could still serve as the source of reproductive materials. It might be possible to take an egg from a woman who has died, then have it fertilized immediately by a spouse, relative, or lover and frozen. It might also be possible to remove ovaries from a deceased person and transplant them to another person, to a uterus, or to both. The appeal to personal autonomy and free choice provides no answers to what ethical values and rules ought to guide the use of these technological possibilities.

PARENTING THROUGH TECHNOLOGY TO WIN BIG PRIZES

In January 1996 Mandy Allwood began taking fertility drugs. Three months later, the young Englishwoman found she was pregnant—very pregnant. Her doctor told her that she was carrying eight fetuses.

Allwood apparently had gone on her drug regimen unbeknownst to her on-again, off-again boyfriend, Paul Hogan, who has said that he had a precise memory of the moment of passion that produced Allwood's octuplets. Baby making, he stated, had occupied no place in his lusty thoughts. Allwood had taken up with Hogan even though a doctor had warned her that she should not engage in sex because the drugs had produced far too many fertile eggs. She was indifferent to the fact that Hogan was living with another woman by whom he had sired two children.

When Allwood found out she was carrying eight fetuses, she hired a publicist and sold the story of her miracle to a London trashy tabloid. The publisher promised her that if she gave birth to eight babies and granted the tabloid exclusive rights to their story, she would pocket one million dollars in cash and prizes.

The news media, ever alert since the O. J. Simpson trial to the newsworthiness of stories broken in the tabloids, ran with the story. Headlines, wire stories, and editorials popped up all over the place about the gutty or goofy Brit mum who might make a cool mil and finally lasso her man if she could pop the eight tiny tykes out of the oven.

The problem was that Allwood's decision to go forward with her pregnancy—her free choice—was dangerous for her and lethal for her babies. By trying to deliver eight fetuses she was condemning them all to a certain death. No birth involving eight fetuses has ever produced a viable child. Extreme prematurity and a far-too-early birth is the inevitable result of carrying that many children. And carrying eight fetuses is a grave threat to the health of the mother as well. Indeed, all eight fetuses were delivered prematurely and all died.

Allwood created the moral dilemma of what to do about an octuplet pregnancy when she chose to have sex despite having been warned that her fertility drugs had produced too many eggs. Her doctor contributed to this moral mess when fertility drugs were given to a single woman who already had a son. The media was complicit in fostering terrible consequences from bad choices—and not just the boneheads at the tabloid who offered Allwood a big prize if she would risk her own and her children's death. The media made Allwood into a celebrity even though her motive in deciding to defy the odds was to win a million-dollar prize.

Regulations in the United Kingdom were inadequate for stopping a single fertile mother from using drugs to boost her fertility, having sex with a man with whom she wanted a baby but who had no idea she was trying to boost her fertility, and then compromising her own health and the health of the resulting fetuses by trying to bring them all to term. There are even fewer obstacles to irresponsible choice in the United States.

Respect for choice is an important and core value of reproduction. But it is of little value if the choice is based on deception and is of questionable value if the person making the choices is willing to choose to manipulate medical technology to achieve ends that have nothing to do with the best interest of future lives and everything to do with using the technology to advance individual self-interest.

DESIGNER EMBRYOS

Two distinct genetic markers now exist which are predictive of dispositions to develop breast cancer. The availability of these markers has not escaped the notice of those involved in reproductive technology such as in vitro fertilization. Clinics on both sides of the Atlantic are already offering to screen embryos for the marker for breast cancer. But it certainly is not obvious that the moral thing to do is to offer parents a choice for screening embryos for a disease that will not appear for many decades if at all.

Nor is it in any way obvious what level of risk would merit offering prospective parents a genetic test for a condition or disorder or even what behaviors or traits ought be considered as medically relevant for embryo biopsy. Should parents be the only ones to decide if they think the risk of breast cancer or Alzheimer's or Huntington's disease is worth testing their embryos? Individual choice may be sufficient to resolve issues about whether or not persons would want to know their genetic predispositions and risks. But choice is not sufficient to guide decisions for those who cannot let their wishes and desires be known—the person who will result if particular embryos are used to make a baby. And choice is certainly not sufficient if clinics and companies use the availability of testing to frighten people into believing that if they do not choose to test their embryos for diseases that will not appear for decades if at all, they are irresponsible or bad parents.

Steps to Cope with Technological Wizardry

The most persuasive argument for more oversight with respect to reproductive technology does not stem from anything that has happened in the field but from what is to come. What is sorely missing is an ethic to govern reproductive technology that takes seriously the need for choice to be guided by true informed consent, regulations that require full and accurate disclosure of information about reproductive technologies in a timely and ongoing manner, and regulations that protect the interests of persons who are used to create or are created with the assistance of technology.

The moral principles that ought to govern the use of assisted reproductive technology are not that difficult to locate. If the goal of using technology to help people make babies is to help the infertile have biological offspring, protect the interests and welfare of any children who are created, and ensure the autonomy, dignity, and self-determination of those who use technology to create children, then some simple principles might guide professional conduct and public policy.

Those who use reproductive technology must be permitted to do so in an informed and uncoerced manner. They should know all of their options and choices. No one should become a parent without the person's express consent. Nothing should be done with reproductive materials without the express consent of the parties who created them. Money and commercialism should be kept to a minimum where the creation of life is concerned. Those who use technology to make babies ought to be infertile or face serious risks to their health if they try to have their own children by means of sex and pregnancy. And providers should not utilize technology, even if it is requested, unless they are reasonably certain that any child who is created will have at least one person capable of being a good parent until the child reaches adulthood.

Following these simple moral rules may not seem especially difficult. Nor do the principles seem especially controversial as instrumental to achieving the ends of fulfilling people's wishes to have children in ways consistent with self-determination, dignity, and the best interest of children. But implementing these principles would require a sea change in the practices now followed in assisted reproduction.

To enable true informed consent, those involved in the infertility business must keep records and basic information about their patients, the handling of reproductive materials, and the outcomes of treatment in a standardized, uniform format. They would have to regularly report on the status of stored reproductive materials to the persons from whom they were obtained.

In addition, it is ludicrous to think that true informed consent can be obtained from persons whose financial well-being depends upon attracting customers in an increasingly competitive marketplace. With the appearance of dubious marketing and advertising campaigns, including money-back guarantees and the hyping of unproved procedures and techniques, the market is overwhelming the ability of patients to make truly informed choices.

Advertising and patient recruitment in the making of babies must be subject to tougher standards and control. Periodic inspections of programs and their quality control procedures as well as independent audits of clinic performance should be implemented, preferably under the auspices of a professional society that can then certify and if necessary sanction programs and program directors.

In order to make valid choices, patients have the right to be given complete data disclosure on the outcome of different forms of treatment, by center, by doctor, and involving patients who are comparable in health and age. These numbers should provide comparisons to untreated populations in terms of pregnancies and births among those who do not continue their infertility care, since some percentage of the conceptions and births attributed to infertility treatment is the result of natural forms of conception that are not aggressively detected by current data-collection methods in the fertility industry. Those who have stored gametes or embryos should be given periodic updates as to their status with requests for instruction from donors as to their disposition.

Clinics ought to be held to minimal, enforceable performance standards. They should be using standardized consent forms that are designed with patient input and subject to periodic updating and review. Fertility programs should also make their policies concerning eligibility for treatment known, and these should be subject to periodic review and modification as well as a condition of certification. Standardized follow-up of those who make gametes available, of those who take infertility treatment, and of at least some representative cohort of children who are conceived with technological assistance should be a requirement for reimbursement by public or private sources.

These minimal steps are necessary simply to enhance the ability of individuals to make informed, voluntary choices. But they are not sufficient. Society needs to create public and private forums where the thorny challenges raised by advances in reproductive technology can be aired, debated, then translated into legislation if necessary.

It is scandalous that the United States still has not made any policy decisions about the control and custody of human reproductive materials and embryos. This failure is especially shocking because in a number of cases disputes have broken out between those who have created embryos and the providers of infertility services over who "owns" or controls embryos. The relationship between genetics, gestation, and parenting in setting the terms of control and custody of children must be thought through and not left to the vagaries of individual clinic policies or allowed to be settled by the person who has the most resources to bring to bear in a legal battle.

Similarly, policy decisions need to be made about the requirements and conditions that should govern the creation of a baby. The easiest way to see why this is so is to compare the steps necessary to become involved in an adoption, with home visits and parental screening, and in reproductive technology, where babies are available simply to the highest bidder. At a minimum, policies must be put in place stating who can use reproductive technologies, including statements about age, the existence of infertility, and the need for a stable, psychologically fit parent or parents.

There is no excuse for the cavalier attitude U.S. society continues to tolerate about how babies are made. Keeping matters in the hands of the private sector with desperate persons left to their own devices and resources does no service to the infertile and risks the well-being of children. The right to reproduce is not a right to be exploited; nor is it a right that extends to the creation of children in a moral and legal thicket where their interests and society's obligation to protect those interests are ignored. The free market is a dangerous, costly environment for making babies; caveat emptor is not a sufficient ethic to guide the creation of new lives.

two

The Intrusion of Evil: The Use of Data from Unethical Medical Experiments

SHOULD THOSE WORKING TODAY in the biomedical sciences make use of information obtained by unethical means? Some dismiss this question as too rare to be worthy of serious discussion. Ruling out the question as not needing an answer reflects either defensiveness or naiveté. To ask whether information acquired by immoral means ought to be used does not imply that the practice is so corrupt that the question cannot be avoided. The question of whether or not data obtained through immoral conduct ought to be preserved, referenced, cited, taught, and applied in the classroom or clinic simply reflects the truth that immoral conduct and inhumane experiments are a part, albeit a small part, of science.

In 1993, a special panel convened by the National Academy of Sciences published the results of an inquiry into a series of experiments involving the testing of chemical weapons. The panel found that from 1942 to 1975 tens of thousands of United States military personnel were subjected to chemical weapons experiments without their consent. The panel concluded that the experiments clearly violated the rights of those who were the subjects:

... the treatment and care of W.W. II chemical warfare production workers and the conduct of later military experiments with human subjects . . . demonstrated a well-ingrained pattern of abuse and neglect. Although the human subjects were called "volunteers" it was clear from the official reports that recruitment of the W.W. II human subjects as well as many of those in later experiments was accomplished through lies and half-truths. (Pechura and Rall, 1993, p. vii).

Some of those who "volunteered" died prematurely. Others were left with severe disabilities.

While the experiments have now been recognized as manifestly immoral, the fact remains that much of what is known about the health effects of chemical weapons such as mustard gas is based on this research. The studies derived from the experiments are cited and referenced in many textbooks, reports, and journals in a wide variety of fields. Regimes such as Saddam Hussein's in Iraq have manufactured and used chemical weapons against both military and civilian targets. During the Gulf War the Iraqis deployed chemical weapons and were apparently prepared to use them. If immoral studies are the only source of information about the effects of some forms of lethal chemical weapons, should this information be used?

It is sometimes argued that the question of using information from unethical experiments merits a simple answer—no. Good science and good ethics must go hand in hand. Valid information cannot be derived from situations in which subjects are misled, abused, or mistreated (Pozos in Caplan, 1992c).

Such a view ignores the historical fact that useful information can be obtained under the most morally heinous circumstances. Revelations concerning the exposure of military personnel, miners, prisoners, mentally retarded children in institutions, and unsuspecting patients in hospitals to clandestine research involving the use of toxic and radioactive substances shows that immoral research and useful, valuable data can go hand in hand (Advisory Committee, 1995).

No research findings, however, demonstrate the dilemma of what to do with tainted data so clearly as the experiments and studies conducted by German scientists on concentration camp inmates during the Second World War. These horrid experiments present a terrible legacy of scientific data and information smeared with suffering and death.

More than two dozen different research projects were undertaken in camps at Dachau, Auschwitz, and Ravensbruck. German physicians and researchers studied such topics as the effect of high-altitude decompression on the human body, the efficacy of sulfanilamide for treating gunshot wounds, the utility of electroshock treatment, the impact of stress on menstruation and ovulation, and the physiological response of the human body to extreme cold (Caplan, 1992c). Other studies were undertaken at a number of institutes and universities of the tissues, bodies, and brains of twins, dwarves, the mentally ill, and those with congenital defects who were killed in various camps in order to understand the genetics, physiology, and anatomy of these disorders and conditions. The products of Nazi horror found their way into tissue collections, anatomy texts, and registries of birth defects and anomalies (Wade, 1996).

Some of those involved in doing research in the camps were manifestly inept or incompetent. Physicians such as Josef Mengele indulged their personal pet theories of biology and conducted barbarous, bizarre experiments on children and women of no possible scientific merit. Their subjects were almost always sick, starving, and uncooperative. But it is not possible to dismiss all of the experimentation and investigation that the Nazis carried out as bad science performed by incompetents on the fringe. Some of the findings of Nazi science were deemed useful and important by a number of governments, including the British, U.S., Soviet, and Japanese governments, at the end of the war. Indeed, the studies done with obvious military application were seen as so useful that those who conducted them became the objects of a fierce struggle as part of the spoils of war. Information from the studies found its way into numerous classified government reports. Some findings were channeled into the literature of biomedical science where they continue to be cited to the present day.

Citations to the Nazi research on hypothermia can be found in medical journals and textbooks throughout the postwar decades (Pross, 1992). Nazi research on exposure to phosgene gas and on the impact of stress on menstruation has been cited by U.S. researchers during the past ten years in both mainstream biomedical journals and government reports (Sun, 1988). Other work undertaken in the concentration camps in areas as wide-ranging as genetics, anatomy, anthropology, and endocrinology continues to appear in medical schools and medical journals.

One reason why the issue of tainted data has occasioned relatively little comment is that if information generated under such awful circumstances as a Dachau or a Natzweiler is cited, then presumably any information, no matter how despicable or abusive its origins, will be used in science and medicine. If even the circumstances of the Holocaust do not suffice to place research findings off limits, what circumstances would?

The mere existence of data, even important and unique data, need not compel its acceptance into biomedical science. Many medical and scientific journals such as the *New England Journal of Medicine* and the

Journal of the American Medical Association have adopted a policy of not publishing findings if the research that produces the data is not conducted in compliance with existing federal requirements governing human (and animal) experimentation.

It should be a standard policy for all journals, textbooks, and professional publications that new data must be generated by moral means in order to be published. This policy would commit the biomedical community to the view that even if good science and good ethics do not always go hand in hand, it is the obligation of the biomedical community to see that only research conducted in compliance with minimal moral standards of research is published. The adoption of such a policy would go a long way toward showing younger scientists and students that in the race to acquire new knowledge, the ethical treatment of subjects must take first priority.

Adoption of the principle that newly created data will not be admitted into the realm of science without some demonstration that its creation meets basic expectations about the treatment of human subjects does not, however, help in deciding what to do when data already exists that has been obtained under questionable or obviously immoral circumstances. The fact that Nazi data has been and continues to be used does not end the discussion as to the ethical propriety of continuing to use this information. Even if one holds the view that once information exists, no matter how tainted, there is no real, practical choice about whether or not to use it, the question of how and with what restrictions the data can be used still must be faced. The moral challenge of how to handle existing tainted data is not confined to the barbarities of the Nazis.

Issues concerning how to use information that already exists and has become a part of medicine are poignantly raised by the most notorious example of immoral research in the United States in this century—the Tuskegee study. In 1932, the Public Health Service began a study involving hundreds of poor black men living near Tuskegee, Alabama, who were infected with syphilis. The goal of the study was to understand the natural history of the disease. Subjects were recruited to participate in the study with false promises of treatment. During the forty years that the study ran, informed consent was never obtained. Even when penicillin became available in the late 1940s, it was not offered to the study subjects (Jones, 1981). Indeed, the subjects were actually deceived and given placebo treatments rather than penicillin.

Despite the immorality of the Tuskegee study, its findings play a central role in the contemporary understanding of the symptoms and course of syphilis. What physicians and public health officials know about syphilis is so strongly rooted in the findings of the Tuskegee study that, short of throwing all books on venereal and infectious diseases out of the libraries of the world, there is no way to avoid citing, referencing, and talking about the study.

Anyone who doubts the ubiquity of the Tuskegee findings in today's medicine need only duplicate my own research. A random survey of medical textbooks and peer-reviewed journals published during the past ten years in one medical school library turned up four explicit references to the study's findings in textbooks and eight other direct references to the Tuskegee study findings in the journals. None of these references were accompanied by any discussion of the moral abuses that characterized the Tuskegee study or the legacy of protections for human subjects that the forty-year study spawned (Caplan, 1992b).

The unethical Tuskegee study, by the reactions it caused, became the source of most of the existing protections created for human subjects in the United States. But despite its notoriety, it has not proved to be an incentive for the creation of policies or rules on handling data obtained by immoral means.

Echoes of Tuskegee can be found in other long-term studies of disease. Much of what is known about exposure to intense amounts of radiation comes from long-term follow-up studies on those who survived the atomic bomb blasts at Hiroshima and Nagasaki. The Japanese view these epidemiological reports with very mixed feelings. Many feel the innocent victims of war continue to be exploited by those who caused them grievous injury (Lindee, 1995).

Similarly, some of what is known about the effects of radon on the human body comes from monitoring conducted by the United States government of Navajo miners in the southwestern United States in the 1950s and 1960s. Native Americans take little solace in the fact that much valuable information on the dangers of radon has been reaped from the surreptitious study of men whom the government knew to be doing especially dangerous work but who were never told (Samet et al., 1984; Advisory Committee on Human Radiation Experiments, 1995) of the dangers their government knew they faced.

When data has been acquired by immoral means or under immoral circumstances it is often too late to talk of ignoring or excising it from biomedicine. I know of no case in which data known to have been produced by immoral means has been banned or eliminated from medicine. The desire to know once the data has been created simply overwhelms the need to honor those from whom the data was obtained.

The question of whether to use what has not already been cited and, if so, how, continues to loom over biomedicine. The abuse of human subjects for reasons of national security has recently presented biomedicine with another moral conundrum. German scientists, with the support of the German government, are beginning the process of analyzing a huge archive of meticulous medical records on 450,000 workers who were exposed to various levels of radiation. The exposure took place over the past forty years while the workers were mining and processing uranium as part of the former East German government's secret program to supply the Soviet Union with weapons-grade material for making atomic bombs (Kahn, 1993).

Scientists around the world are eager to see what the data reveal about the effects of regular exposure over many years to low levels of radiation, radioactive dust, and radon as well as various combinations of radiation and toxic chemicals. A U.S. expert believes that the archive will be extremely valuable "not only in [understanding radiation exposure] in mining populations but also how it translates into [understanding exposure to] domestic radon. . . ." One scientist describes the archive as "the world's biggest treasure chest of data on radiation and human health" (Kahn, 1993, 448). It is an especially grisly treasure chest. According to records which became available with the collapse of the East German regime in 1989, at least 20,000 workers died from lung disease associated with exposure to radiation and radioactive dust. Thousands more will certainly die in the years to come.

And the dilemmas raised by tainted knowledge acquired during the Cold War will not end with the East German atomic bomb effort. All over the former Soviet Union and Eastern Europe hundreds of thousands of people have been exposed to the effects of toxic substances, unsafe nuclear power plants such as Chernobyl, and pollutants generated by regimes that put national security ahead of public health. Biomedicine will soon confront a grim epidemiological bonanza as the innocent victims of these policies sicken and die.

It still isn't known what sort of research—medical, psychological, behavioral—organizations such as the CIA and the FBI engaged in in the midst of the battle between East and West. But locked in the archives of these organizations are likely to be findings of keen interest to those who want to understand everything from the power of behavioral conditioning to the medical consequences of torture.

The issue of whether tainted data should be used seems beyond debate. When even minimal stakes are involved, data is used. The only issue still open for debate is whether those who find themselves either analyzing data acquired through immoral conduct or who cite or reference such work bear some obligation to convey the taint which clings to it. Can any rules for the handling of tainted data be promulgated?

First, there is an obligation to see whether the tainted data is the only possible source of information. When alternatives exist, they ought to be used. There is no excuse for the invocation of data acquired immorally unless it is the only possible source.

Second, those who use obviously tainted data have a duty to make sure that the goal or purpose for which the data is being used is of vital importance. Using data acquired through torture or the abuse of human subjects to advance a commercial goal does not square with the overarching importance of making sure that those who conduct research understand their responsibilities to subjects.

Third, whenever space permits, most especially in review articles and textbooks, some comment must be made about the circumstances under which the tainted data was obtained. And finally, some attempt should be made, when circumstances permit, to discuss the use of tainted data with the subjects involved in its creation in order to ensure that the policies for the use of the information take into account their preferences and that they understand why and how such information will be used.

Unethical conduct can produce data of value to science. There is no avoiding this fact. This reality confronts the biomedical and research communities with a moral challenge that has not been adequately addressed by policy or professional guidelines.

Should new knowledge acquired by immoral means be treated as taboo and kept outside the domain of mainstream science? It should. This means that editors and peer reviewers of journals and periodicals must agree that they will not permit the publication of data, regardless of its value or importance, if it has been obtained by immoral means, including a lack of explicit informed consent or in circumstances such as the torture of political prisoners or prisoners of war where consent is obviously impossible (Angell, 1992).

When data already exists and has somehow entered the domain of science, a number of simple moral principles should guide its use. Involvement, when possible, of the actual subjects used to create the suspect data in decisions about its release and use should be obligatory. Those seeking to cite or invoke tainted data should understand that it must be put to use for an important purpose, that no alternatives are available, and that the circumstances surrounding the creation of the data must be explicitly acknowledged. Investigators who fail to follow ethical requirements for research should not receive credit or acknowledgment in the presentation or referencing of tainted data.

If it is neither prudent nor possible to turn away from that which is already known, regardless of how it came to be known, then the biomedical community must be clear about the responsibilities and duties of those who use such data. Future generations of researchers must see that it is good ethics, not just good data, that really matters.

three

Have a Heart?
The Ethical Lessons of
the Development of the
Total Artificial Heart

Early History

IN 1964, THE UNITED STATES CONGRESS budgeted $581,000 to establish an artificial heart program at the National Institutes of Health (NIH). This was the first large-scale effort by any nation to support systematic research into the development of an artificial heart. The effort to build a reliable, totally implantable artificial heart has still not succeeded. Even though the device does not yet exist, however, the artificial heart has been at the center of a heated ethical, economic, and policy debate about the merits of building such a device since the 1960s. The discussion of the wisdom of the project has also served as a paradigm for debating the future of expensive technologies in the U.S. health care system.

Scientists and physicians in many countries have dreamed for centuries of curing fatal forms of heart disease by creating a mechanical substitute. As recently as the 1950s, most physicians and engineers thought there were too many technical and design problems to undertake the creation of an implantable mechanical heart. But technological advances during the 1960s in engineering fields such as metallurgy, fluid dynamics, electronics, and computer modeling made some scientists think that its construction might actually be possible. The emergence of the kidney dialysis machine, which could mimic the functions of a human kidney, created a fundamental change in attitude in medicine about the feasibility of building an artificial heart.

Constructing an artificial heart requires materials such as metals, ceramics, plastics, and polymers that are lightweight and durable. At the same time, these materials must be biologically inert. They must not trigger attacks by the body's natural system of immune defenses that would lead to the disruption of the circulatory system and, ultimately, death. An artificial heart also requires sufficiently smooth surfaces so as not to disrupt blood flow through the heart or permit damage to fragile blood cells. A total artificial heart (TAH) needs a power source that can maintain a steady stream of energy for long periods while being small enough to fit completely inside the body. Both the pump and the power source must be capable of responding to changes in position, temperature, and pressure associated with the needs of the person using the machine.

The decision to launch a program to try to build a totally implantable heart had its roots in a series of exploratory meetings during the 1950s at the NIH (Shaw, 1984). Enthusiasm for undertaking the research accelerated in the 1960s as physicians and engineers began to build and successfully use the first heart-lung machine, an external pump that could be used to support blood circulation in the body. After a few hours' use, the machine damaged the blood cells. But crude as it was, it did inspire physicians and engineers to think that perhaps a permanent device was not beyond their reach.

As the U.S. space program began to enjoy success, optimism grew in both scientific and government circles about the feasibility of taking on large-scale technological challenges. Many officials in government were impressed with the productive results that the space program and the military secured from centrally funded, programmatic research. Workers in medicine and biomedical science saw themselves as being able to overcome the many technical obstacles through hard work, directed budgets, and targeted programs. The space program had as its goal putting a man on the moon before the end of the 1960s. The artificial heart program launched at the National Institutes of Health in 1964 set as its goal the testing of a total artificial heart in a human being by

Valentine's Day, 1970 (Bernstein, 1984). Ever since, there has been an artificial heart program at the NIH as part of what is now the National Heart, Lung, and Blood Institute with a budget of at least $10 million per year.

The goal of implanting an artificial heart by the end of the 1960s was not attained. A major hurdle was the development of an energy source capable of providing long-term power to an artificial heart that could fit inside the body. Not only was progress slow but, during the time artificial heart researchers were trying to overcome the large number of technical challenges that confronted them, a new alternative to the mechanical heart appeared—cardiac transplantation. On December 3, 1967, Dr. Christiaan N. Barnard, using an organ obtained from a cadaver, performed the first heart transplant in a human being at Groote Schuur Hospital in Cape Town, South Africa. Although Barnard's patient survived for only eighteen days, the prospect of transplanting hearts from cadavers somewhat diminished interest in medical and government circles in the artificial heart.

In 1969, Dr. Denton Cooley implanted a crude mechanical heart in a human recipient at Baylor University College of Medicine, but most of the device, including the power source, remained outside the body. Cooley stated that his sole motive for using this primitive, untested device was the desperate hope that it might help a dying patient live until a donor heart became available for transplant. This attempt was executed without the approval of Cooley's superiors or any government agency. The recipient, Haskell Karp, died shortly after the implant.

Cooley's actions set off a storm of controversy within his medical center. Karp's wife later decided to file suit against Dr. Cooley for failure to obtain proper informed consent to the experiment. Texas courts held that since the procedure was experimental, there were no agreed-upon informed-consent standards that governed artificial heart implant surgery and dismissed the suit.

In the late 1960s, the idea of using atomic power to run a TAH gained favor. Some researchers thought that a small implantable capsule of plutonium could be used. The Artificial Heart Assessment Panel, specially convened by the NIH, concluded in 1973 that while the "advent of the totally implantable artificial heart" would be "an earthshaking event," the use of atomic power posed the possibility of unacceptable radiation exposure risks to the public health (National Heart and Lung Institute, 1973).

As continuing problems with materials and limited success in animal studies spawned more doubts, James Shannon, then director of the NIH, decided in 1973 to change the mission of the federal government's artificial heart program. Instead of being aimed at the construction of a TAH, federal funds would be directed toward the design, construction, and testing of a partial artificial heart, the left-ventricular assist device (LVAD).

The left chamber or ventricle of the human heart does the greatest share of the work of circulating blood through the body. Heart attacks and other forms of heart disease frequently damage this portion of the heart. An LVAD is a pump capable of supplementing the function of the left ventricle to allow a weakened or damaged heart to support life. It requires no implantable power source and its design can be simpler, since it does not have to duplicate all of the functions of a heart for prolonged periods.

For the next fifteen years, the NIH spent approximately $10 million a year on research on LVADs. By the early 1990s a number of universities and private companies were undertaking clinical trials of LVADs in the United States and other nations. A small amount of work on the TAH continued outside the United States, but support for this research came almost entirely from private funds.

The Private Sector

In 1967, Dr. Willem Kolff, the inventor of an early prototype of an artificial kidney dialysis machine, which he built in Holland during the Nazi occupation, moved to the University of Utah in Salt Lake City. His work on the dialysis machine led him to believe that it might be possible to build a mechanical heart. Over the next ten years, he assembled a large interdisciplinary team of medical, veterinary, and engineering researchers, among whom were the physicians Clifford Kwan-Gett and Robert Jarvik.

In the early 1970s, Kwan-Gett and later Jarvik began testing mechanical hearts in sheep and calves. These hearts fit inside the body of the animal but used an external air compressor powered by electricity provided from a wall outlet to create the force necessary to circulate blood. The Kwan-Gett artificial heart was made of plastic with carefully designed internal surfaces to minimize the danger of damage to blood cells caused by the machine's pumping action. In 1974, what had become known as the Jarvik-3 model kept a calf alive for three months.

In 1976, Kolff and some of his Utah colleagues formed a private company, Kolff Medical Associates, to attract venture capital to support their research. In order to interest private investors, they had to create a marketing program for their mechanical heart. The decision to proceed with a private company constituted a first step into the emerging and often ethically controversial world of public-private partnerships intended to advance medical research.

After further testing and redesign of the Jarvik heart, Kolff's research team managed to use a Jarvik-7 to keep animals alive for as long as eight months. Kolff Medical Associates applied in 1980 for permission from the University of Utah Medical Center human experimentation committee—or, as it is also known, the institutional review board or IRB—to try the device on a human being. The group also sought permission from the Food and Drug Administration, which, since late 1976, had had authority for regulating the testing and marketing of medical devices. While awaiting approval, members of the Utah artificial heart group traveled to Philadelphia and conducted a series of three practice implants of a Jarvik-7 heart on brain-dead patients at Temple University Medical Center. Permission to use the cadavers was obtained from family members by Jack Kolff, Willem Kolff's son, then a surgeon at Temple.

After many weeks of resubmissions and revisions, the IRB at Utah and the FDA granted approval to undertake a series of seven implants of a Jarvik-7 heart in human beings at the University of Utah. Kolff and Jarvik, who had renamed their company Symbion, selected a young surgeon, Dr. William DeVries, to perform the first implant in a human recipient.

Initially the Utah group thought it would try the device on patients who encountered life-threatening problems while undergoing heart surgery. Sometimes during a heart operation surgeons find that their patient's heart is so severely damaged that they cannot "wean," or remove, the patient from a heart-lung machine without causing the patient's immediate death. The Symbion researchers argued (and the IRB accepted) the view that since persons who could not be weaned from heart-lung machines were doomed to die, they constituted an appropriate pool of people to approach for permission to try out the Jarvik-7 device. A few patients who had severe heart disease were asked about their willingness to be put on a Jarvik heart if they could not be weaned from life-support during surgery. A small number agreed to an implant if life-threatening problems developed during their heart operations, but all were able to be safely taken off life-support after surgery.

DeVries and his colleagues then revised their research protocol to expand the pool of possible subjects to include patients with very severe, life-threatening congestive heart failure resulting from cardiomyopathy, a mysterious condition that causes irreversible, fatal damage to the muscle of the heart. This change was approved by the IRB in May 1982.

Barney B. Clark, a retired dentist who had been admitted to the University of Utah Medical Center on November 29, 1982, with cardiomyopathy, was deemed to be an "ideal candidate" for the first implant of the Jarvik heart (Fox and Swazey, 1992). He signed the eighteen-page consent form the night he was admitted to the hospital. When his heart began to fail on December 1, he was taken to the operating room and, after a nine-hour operation, became the first human being to receive an artificial heart as a permanent replacement for his own.

The Clark experiment attracted the most media attention in the history of human experimentation. Jarvik and DeVries as well as other University of Utah officials spent countless hours speaking with the media about the operation, the device, and Dr. Clark's health status. In the days after the implant, the health care team made many optimistic pronouncements about Clark's chances for survival. Clark, however, underwent a very rocky course over the 112 days he lived with the Jarvik-7 device. He suffered a wide range of complications that resulted in three additional surgical procedures. After a few weeks on the machine, his emotional and cognitive state deteriorated severely. On more than one occasion he asked that the artificial heart be turned off. This was not done. He lingered on the machine in an unconscious state for many days. More than 1,300 persons, including political figures, members of the governing council of the Mormon Church of which Clark was a member, many of his doctors, and media representatives from around the world, attended his funeral in Seattle.

The Clark experiment was pronounced a success by DeVries and the Utah group. They had kept alive a man in the final stages of heart failure for well over three months. The IRB at Utah, however, was troubled by the many complications that had arisen during the experiment. They asked for many changes and clarifications in the research protocol before giving DeVries permission to try another implant.

The Clark experiment raises many troubling questions about the adequacy of informed consent on the part of those who have received artificial hearts. It also highlights moral quandaries that surround research on anyone suffering from a terminal illness.

Can those facing certain death really be said to exercise informed consent? It is hard to imagine how, since the very fact of imminent death limits the realities of choice to doing anything that a physician offers as holding any hope. If true consent requires a balanced presentation of the risks and benefits involved, can a person who is both researcher and therapist be the source? Those conducting the research on the total artificial heart were so enthusiastic and hopeful about its prospects and saw their careers and financial futures as so intimately tied to the device that they could not possibly have provided a realistic picture of the risks and dangers inherent in the experiment (Fox and Swazey, 1992). Not only are the circumstances of terminal illness inherently coercive, it is impossible for the dying to hear anything but good news from researchers who have every imaginable reason to offer it.

Controversies also swirled around the issue of ownership of the stock of Symbion, how best to find sources to pay for the next implant (Barney Clark's bill exceeded $250,000), and how to finance the research. Insurance companies do not like to pay for new and experimental treatments. The cost of such procedures must come from research grants or simply be assumed by the institution where the experiments are being done.

On July 31, 1984, DeVries abruptly brought the controversies to a halt. He announced at a press conference that he and the artificial heart program had left Salt Lake City and would begin work immediately at the Humana Hospital Audubon in Louisville, Kentucky. Thus, much to the amazement of his colleagues at Utah, DeVries very quickly moved himself and his family to a large, private hospital thousands of miles away.

Humana Audubon was part of a corporation that was trying to establish itself as a national leader in the for-profit health care sector. One principle owner of the company, David Jones, pledged to DeVries that the company was willing to underwrite the costs of "up to 100 implants" if he would move his artificial heart program to Louisville. DeVries, angry at what he saw as "red tape" and "bureaucracy" holding up his research at Utah as well as at criticism over the fact that he held stock in Symbion, jumped at the chance.

During the next three years, from 1984 to 1987, four more hearts were implanted as permanent replacements. William J. Schroeder, who received his implant of a Jarvik heart on November 29, 1984, underwent surgery in Louisville less than two months after the IRB at Humana Audubon had been asked to give its approval. Schroeder initially did well on the heart, but he suffered a stroke within nineteen days. During the next 620 days he spent on the device, he had three more strokes, the last of which brought about his death. The other recipients of these primitive total artificial hearts—two at Louisville, one in Sweden, and one in Arizona—experienced equally rocky courses and ultimately died. It became clear from these experiments that the Jarvik-7 was not suitable for use as a permanent replacement device.

In January 1988, the new director of the National Heart, Lung, and Blood Institute, Dr. Claude Lenfant, decided to cancel the NIH program to build a TAH. He felt that the recent experience with artificial hearts clearly indicated that the best use of such devices would be to assist failing hearts to buy time until a transplant could be found. Lenfant argued that a totally implantable artificial heart was still at least ten years away and might well wind up benefiting a relatively small number of patients at great cost. However, the threat to shut down research on the TAH created a whirlwind of protest in Congress. Legislators in states such as Utah and Massachusetts, where heart research was being conducted, fought to block Lenfant's plan. By the end of 1988, $20 million was awarded to four centers to continue this research.

On January 11, 1990, the FDA withdrew its approval for the clinical testing of Jarvik-7 devices in human beings, citing concerns about the safety of the device and the quality control of the manufacturer, Symbion. In July 1991, the National Academy of Sciences' Institute of Medicine issued a study that recommended continued federal funding for both LVADs and TAHs. The study predicted that a reliable LVAD would become available in the late 1990s and a TAH by around 2005 (Institute of Medicine, 1991). Federal funding for research on both permanent and temporary artificial hearts has continued.

Ethics and Mechanical Hearts

A number of ethical concerns are raised by the history of total-artificial-heart research and use. Three issues stand out as especially important, both in analyzing what took place in Utah and Kentucky and what might happen in the future: the ethics of innovative experimentation involving human subjects, the benefits alleged to be associated with the temporary use of an artificial heart or other new form of therapy, and fairness in the allocation of scarce new forms of life-saving technologies. These issues are specific to the artificial heart and, moreover, apply generally to all forms of new and expensive, high-technology health care.

HUMAN EXPERIMENTATION

Two sorts of protection exist for persons who participate in medical research: informed consent and review of research proposals by local committees of scientists (IRBs). The adequacy of both protections is called into question by what happened to those who served as the first subjects in whom total artificial hearts were used in the 1980s.

The subjects, Barney Clark, William Schroeder, Murray Hayden, and the rest, were in extremely vulnerable circumstances. They faced certain death if the device was not used. For some of these men the recognition that they were dying had come suddenly and unexpectedly. For all, the complexities of the implant, the surgery, and the rigorous postimplant monitoring of the device were extremely intimidating.

Subjects heard about the possible risks and benefits of the experimental surgery only from researchers who had a powerful interest in wanting their work to proceed. There has been a strong conflict of interest on the part of physicians seeking subjects to receive artificial hearts, since they have always acted in the roles of both clinician and researcher for recipients of the device.

The dual role of researcher and clinician is one that is so rife with conflict that it makes sense to take steps to minimize it. Certainly providing patients with access to persons with no direct professional or financial stake in the outcome of new forms of research is essential if anything even vaguely resembling informed consent is to be a feature of research on life-saving therapies.

Not only does the threat of imminent death impair the ability of subjects to make voluntary choices; those charged with reviewing requests to use artificial hearts on institutional review boards have faced serious moral challenges as well. Enormous pressure characterized the race to be the first to use a mechanical heart or to be the first to successfully use one. The financial and publicity stakes involved for the researcher, the institution, and any companies in which the institution or researcher might have an interest were enormous. Local IRBs may not have the requisite expertise or independence to evaluate exactly what sorts of criteria ought to be used to govern subject selection, consent forms, or the methods for accumulating data on subjects over long periods.

TEMPORARY USE

As it became clear in the 1980s that devices then available could not safely support long-term heart function in human beings, artificial hearts were turned to temporary uses. But here too there are tough ethical questions that need to be confronted.

If artificial hearts are to be used on a temporary basis, can they be implanted without the explicit consent of a person who has undergone a sudden, unexpected heart failure? Which patients would constitute the best population for testing devices intended only for temporary use—those nearest to death who made up the population of subjects for permanent implants of Jarvik hearts or those not quite as sick who are most likely to recover if given a respite by an LVAD or temporary use of an artificial heart? It is not clear that those who are given artificial hearts or LVADs on a temporary basis understand whether or under what circumstances they have the right to turn off these devices. Nor is it clear that the use of these devices will contribute overall to an increase in the number of lives saved (Annas, 1993). When cadaver hearts are scarce, the use of artificial hearts or bridge devices as a prelude to transplant means only that the identity of those getting a chance at a transplant may change while the overall number of transplants done remains the same (Caplan, 1992a).

Financing

One obvious moral question raised by research to develop an artificial heart is whether developing this device is the best way to spend limited research dollars in terms of meeting the health care needs of Americans or of the world's population as a whole. Artificial heart research is expensive. The costs of doing the first TAH implants ran into the many hundreds of thousands of dollars. Does it make more sense to pursue other options for the treatment of heart disease or even the prevention of heart disease?

Many experts note that a fully perfected TAH would be likely to cost this nation billions of dollars. Yet those most likely to benefit from access to such a device might be restricted only to those who could afford insurance to pay for mechanical hearts. There are obvious problems of equity and justice in asking all Americans to bear the cost of research for a device that would only be available to some. Questions of fairness also shape any decision to build a machine which may add years of life to those at the end of the life span when there are tens of millions of persons around the globe who die before reaching adolescence from preventable causes of disease and injury. Health policy discussions have not defined and continue to avoid any explicit discussion of how best to allocate resources to perfect new therapies. Dollars still flow toward those diseases for whom advocates and surrogates can clamor the loudest. As the sad legacy of the artificial heart shows, it would be prudent to make considerations of fairness a more central part of this crucial policy debate.

four

"What a Long, Strange Trip It's Been": The Debate over the Use of Fetal Tissue for Transplantation Research

ONE OF PRESIDENT BILL CLINTON'S FIRST acts upon assuming office in his first term was to rescind a ban the Bush administration had imposed in 1988 on the use of federal funds to pay for research on transplants using fetal tissue. The answer to why this narrow area of biomedical research commanded the attention of two presidents reveals the ways in which ethics and politics intertwine in biomedicine.

The controversy over the use of tissue from aborted fetuses for transplantation research was one of the strangest in the annals of human experimentation ethics. The debate focused almost exclusively on the proposals of a tiny handful of scientists in the United States to use fetal tissue transplants to see whether they might be of benefit to persons suffering from Parkinsonism or diabetes. Opponents of such research protested vehemently that it was immoral and barbaric to use fetal tissue in research. They brought enormous pressure on the Bush administration to ban such research. This in turn set off a spirited response from those concerned to defend abortion rights and those who thought they might benefit from fetal transplants. There was little recognition on the part of anyone involved in the fight, which occupied the last two years of the Bush administration, how truly bizarre it was to debate the morality of fetal tissue research given the decades-long history of using tissues from aborted fetuses in many areas of medical research and the ongoing commitment of the federal government to funding such research.

Transplants using tissue from aborted fetuses were hardly unknown in medicine at the time the debate over the morality of fetal tissue transplants erupted in full fury in 1988. The first experiment involving a transplant using tissue from an aborted fetus took place in Italy with a patient suffering from diabetes. The experiment, which did not succeed, was reported in the medical literature in 1928. The first U.S. experiment involving tissue from aborted fetuses, transplanting bits of fetal pancreas in an attempt to treat a person with life-threatening diabetes, took place in 1939. This experiment also failed. At least one form of fetal tissue transplantation, the use of fetal thymus to replace tissue absent in children born without a thymus, had been established as efficacious and therapeutic years before the big debate broke out (Vawter et al., 1990).

By the early 1970s, many transplant experiments using fetal cells in newborn babies had been undertaken. The subjects were children afflicted with a congenital condition known as DiGeorge's syndrome. Babies with this condition are born with weakened immune systems because they lack a functioning thymus.

The results of transplants using fetal tissue that were reported in the medical literature throughout the 1970s and 1980s were very positive. One such study appeared in the peer-reviewed medical literature a year before the Bush administration imposed its ban (Vawter et al., 1990).

For years, researchers in many nations, most notably Sweden but also China, the United Kingdom, Australia, France, Mexico, and Cuba, had been actively engaged in research programs using fetal tissue from aborted fetuses for transplants (Vawter et al., 1990). If anything, Americans were rather late in pursuing transplantation research compared with scientists in other parts of the world.

Not only did transplants using tissue from electively aborted fetuses have a long history in medicine prior to the Bush administration's ban on federal funding, but fetal tissue from aborted fetuses had long been used in medical research for purposes such as toxicity studies, research on fetal development, and the culturing of tissue lines for all manner of genetic and biological research. These types of experiments continued with federal support throughout the time when the government ban on federal funds for fetal tissue research was imposed. In 1988, the year the ban was imposed, the National Institutes of Health spent $8.3 million on non-transplant-related research involving human fetal tissue.

Not only did the government support research using fetal tissue; the government had historically been involved in procuring such tissue. In 1961, the federal government helped create a tissue bank, the Laboratory for the Study of Human Embryos and Fetuses at the University of Washington, for distributing fetal tissues to researchers in the United States. A similar bank had been in existence in the United Kingdom under the auspices of the British Medical Research Council since 1957. Incredibly, arguments about the ethics of allowing fetal tissue transplant research to proceed were treated as somehow independent from and unconnected to the use of fetal tissue from aborted fetuses for other forms of scientific research which continued with government support throughout the five years the ban existed.

There is only one reason why the nation's leaders, interest groups, members of the media, and scientific societies could find themselves embroiled in a debate about the moral permissibility of research that had a half-century history in medicine, had already proved successful in the treatment of at least one disease, and had used precisely the same source of tissue as many other forms of publicly funded research: politics, specifically, abortion politics. The debate about the use of fetal tissue for transplants was nothing more than a chapter in the nation's long-running debate about the morality of elective abortion (Vawter and Caplan, 1992).

Those who opposed the use of fetal tissue for transplantation built their case around three arguments (Bopp and Burtchaell, 1988). First, if fetal tissue from elective abortions were used in transplantation research, then women might be swayed or motivated to have abortions. Second, if fetal tissue were used in transplantation research, the demand for such tissue might well trigger a market for fetal tissue, leading to more abortions. And third, the use of fetal tissue for transplants would bring moral legitimacy to the practice of abortion—a legitimacy which opponents of elective abortion found unacceptable and deeply troubling. As Dr. Louis W. Sullivan said in announcing his decision to extend the ban on federal funding of human fetal tissue transplantation research despite the recommendation of a special advisory committee to the NIH that the ban be lifted, "one must accept the likelihood that permitting the human fetal research at issue will increase the incidence of abortion across the country" (letter to Dr. William Raub, Acting Director, NIH, November 2, 1989).

Defenders of the use of fetal tissue in the scientific community did not engage these claims about the impact of fetal tissue transplant research upon abortion. They argued, along with many patient advocacy groups, that to prohibit federal funding for fetal tissue research would mean denying hundreds of thousands of Americans their only hope of finding a cure for a host of disabling and life-threatening diseases for which no cures existed (Consultants to the Advisory Committee to the Director, NIH, 1988). The benefits to be garnered from this form of research outweighed any moral reservations about the source of the tissue involved.

This emphasis on the benefits to be gained from permitting fetal tissue transplant research to proceed had the effect of legitimizing concerns that such research would lead to increases in elective abortions. The more one side emphasized the potential benefits to be gained, the more legitimate the concerns seemed of those worried about the need to obtain more tissue to allow transplants to be available to all in need. The scientific and patient advocacy communities appeared to be saying that the benefits to be gained for those with incurable illnesses would outweigh any moral price associated with an increase in abortions.

An NIH advisory committee that looked at the question of federal funding at the request of the director of the NIH spent all of its time and energy considering the impact the funding would have on the incidence of abortion (Consultants to the Advisory Committee to the Director, NIH, 1988). The recommendations which the advisory committee provided in advocating that the research proceed, recommendations which made their way into the congressional legislation enacted in 1993 to regulate fetal transplantation research, strove to ensure that continued funding would not result in an increase in abortions. In taking this focus, the NIH advisory panel gave further credibility to worries about increases in elective abortion rates following in the wake of federally sponsored fetal tissue transplant research.

The strangest thing about the many strange things which characterized the debate about the use of fetal tissue from elective abortions for transplants was that hardly anyone challenged the underlying notion that allowing research on fetal tissue transplants would increase the incidence of abortions (Vawter et al., 1990; Garry, Caplan et al., 1992). There was no evidence then and there is none now that the expenditure of federal funds on other forms of research using fetal tissue from elective abortion has had any impact on rates of abortion. Nor was there any evidence presented that women thinking about or seeking abortions would assign any weight to considerations about the disposition of fetal remains postabortion in deciding whether to carry a pregnancy to term. And no one seemed interested in asking whether the supply of tissue required to conduct a small number of experiments would require more abortions than the one-and-a-half million taking place each year in the United States.

At the time the issue was being debated, a few women came forward in the media claiming that they would impregnate themselves and abort their fetuses to help loved ones who might benefit from fetal tissue transplants. There was no reason to think, however, that their views were in any way typical of women who were actually facing choices about becoming pregnant or having an abortion. Nor was there any scientific reason to believe that directed donation, i.e., picking a particular recipient for tissues or organs, would be any more useful for the purposes of research than using tissues from anonymous random sources. Even if a tiny number of women were willing to conceive in order to generate tissues, there was no reason to think that any of them needed to do this. And there was no reason to believe that researchers would use tissue from a fetus known to have been conceived and aborted solely to generate tissues for research. There was certainly no reason to believe that hordes of women would be motivated to conceive and terminate their pregnancies simply to make tissue available for the purposes of fetal tissue transplant research (Vawter et al., 1991).

If arguments about the motives of women having abortions rested on false assumptions, arguments about markets in fetal tissue rested on ignorance. The sale of human tissue and organs from cadaver sources had been outlawed in the United States for more than fifteen years prior to the ban on federal funding for fetal tissue transplant research. The sale of fetal tissue was specifically outlawed in 1989. The political odds of overturning this ban in order to permit a market in fetal tissue were then and still remain zero (Caplan, 1992a). So concerns that fetal tissue would be bought and sold on the open market had absolutely no foundation, either in the motives that lead women to end pregnancies or in the legal climate of the United States, which would not permit such a market.

These objections, while not really successfully addressed, were not taken all that seriously. Ultimately the argument against providing federal funds for fetal tissue transplant research rested on the issue of the legitimation of abortion. If fetal transplant research were done, would that not make those having abortions feel better about their decisions to end a potential life and thus make abortion morally less repugnant in American society? Those who objected to fetal tissue research really objected to the idea that the use of fetal remains for valuable research might make abortion somewhat less morally problematic for those facing a choice.

The legitimacy claim was the least challenged and the prize winner for least-substantiated of all the ethical objections raised. Women who had abortions would have no way of knowing for certain whether any tissues recovered were actually used in transplantation research. And even if they could find out or knew in a general way that some fetal tissue was used in medical research, why would this knowledge provide solace to women who had doubts about the morality of their choice?

Organs and tissues are taken from the victims of child abuse and murder and are transplanted to others everyday. Lives are saved as a result. Yet the procurement of organs and tissues acquired in the most terrible circumstances has done nothing to change the assessment that society makes of child abuse and murder or those who engage in these behaviors.

Defenders of the use of fetal tissue let all these arguments pass. Their contention was that it made no sense to forgo the great benefits to be had from fetal tissue transplant research for those dying and disabled by incurable diseases. But there was little reason at the time to think that fetal tissue transplant research was anything more than a possibly useful strategy for research. There has been no reason since to change that assessment.

It is not at all clear that fetal tissue transplant research will ever prove helpful in treating human diseases. The state of the science supporting research in this area is highly underdeveloped (Vawter et al., 1990). What is clear is that the moral debate about the use of fetal tissue derived from elective abortions pivoted on arguments based upon assumptions or claims of utility that were at best overblown.

The battle over the use of federal funds for fetal tissue transplant research constituted a case study in how not to hold a moral debate in public. Facts were distorted, made up, or, when inconvenient, ignored. Claims were made about the motives of women that were never rooted in anything other than ideology and bias. Hyped promises about the value of fetal tissue transplant research, research that despite a long history had not shown itself to be any sort of a quick fix for major disabling illnesses and disorders, were allowed to go unchallenged.

It is often said that abortion politics distorts a good deal of U.S. public policy debate. It is often said but rarely explained. The battle of the use of fetal tissue for transplants was a paradigmatic case of how the polemic power of the abortion controversy elevated a minor issue into a national crisis and then allowed it to be resolved with absolutely no connection to history, reality, or fact. Perhaps, at least, there are lessons that can be learned from this debate. Sadly, that does not seem to be true.

In early January 1994, a scientist in Scotland, Roger Gosden of the University of Edinburgh, announced in a story reported in the *New York Times* that he thought it possible to use eggs obtained from aborted fetuses to help infertile women have babies. He said he could do this by harvesting fetal ovaries and grafting them into the ovaries of infertile women. If so, the transplant would be of benefit to women who could not make their own eggs either because they had reached menopause or because they had some disorder or disease that made their eggs abnormal. Gosden said that he had successfully transplanted fetal ovaries in mice and that he would soon be ready to try the technique using human fetal eggs (Kolata, 1994).

It is nothing short of remarkable that a scientist chose to use the lay press to announce findings concerning the harvesting of fetal ovaries. This was not the first time, however, that researchers circumvented the usual channels of peer review with respect to transplants aimed at helping those with incurable diseases. Announcements about the use of adrenal glands and later brain tissue to try to help persons with Parkinsonism using tissue from aborted fetuses had first come to public attention not in articles in scientific journals but in letters to the editor and media reports. While some scientists complain that the media stir the pot of moral controversy concerning scientific advances, it is more often the case, especially in areas pertaining to reproduction, genetic engineering, and the use of fetal tissue, that scientists seek out the media in order to secure further funding, public acclaim, or a demonstration of priority before their work has undergone peer review in the professional literature.

Gosden's announcement met with a storm of controversy. Some commentators in the United Kingdom immediately pronounced the idea of using eggs from aborted fetuses ethically repugnant. A group of British legislators drafted a law, enacted a year later, to outlaw such transplants.

Some ethicists in the United States, including George Annas and Mark Siegler, were quick to condemn the idea as morally suspect. Two members of the medical ethics program at the University of Wisconsin, Alta Charo and Dan Wikler, were so unnerved by the rapid negative reaction to Gosden's claims that they issued a call for a self-imposed moratorium on the proffering of timely opinions about fetal egg harvesting or any advance in reproductive technology (Charo and Wikler, 1994).

Some did not find the idea of harvesting eggs from aborted fetuses so obviously horrible. Nor did they believe, as Charo and Wikler argued, that they ought to muzzle their enthusiasm until a suitable period of deliberative thought had passed.

Professor John Fletcher, a distinguished theologian at the University of Virginia's Program in Biomedical Ethics, acknowledged that taking eggs from aborted fetuses might seem initially bizarre. But, Fletcher maintained, the use of such eggs could help women unable to make eggs to obtain them (Kolata, 1994). Moreover, harvesting eggs from fetuses would reduce the number of women who undergo possibly risky hormonal treatments in order to serve as egg donors. Much as had been argued with respect to the use of fetal tissue for transplants, the benefits of fetal egg transplants ought to outweigh any squeamishness about the source.

Some infertility specialists in the United States declared that those who find the idea of taking eggs from aborted fetuses revolting simply fail to understand the desperation and the anguish of women who desperately want to have a child. The musings of professional worrywarts about the ethics of taking eggs from aborted fetuses pale, these doctors said, in the light of the good that can come from finding a way to allow infertile women to have babies. Consequentialism was used to push aside any moral reservations about the ethics of the means used to reach the consequences.

The proposal to use fetal eggs did not catch on. Opinion, as expressed by politicians, letters to the editor, and statements of professional associations regarding the use of fetal ovaries obtained from aborted fetuses as sources of eggs for the infertile was overwhelmingly negative. This reaction was very different from that which had greeted proposals only six years earlier to use fetal tissue from aborted fetuses for transplant research. Only right-to-life groups seemed to oppose the use of fetal tissue for transplant research, whereas a wide spectrum of individuals evinced concern about the use of fetal eggs and ovaries. Why the difference? Are there any real moral differences between using fetal islet cells to try to control insulin production in a terminally ill diabetic and inserting fetal ovaries taken from the very same aborted fetus for use in a woman whose own ovaries do not function?

There are. Transplanting an islet cell is not the same as transplanting an egg. One procedure might save a life. The other will create a new one. And therein lies a significant moral difference. But before examining the difference it is important to ask whether fetal ovary transplants could really be done.

All of the eggs that a woman will ever have in her life are present by the tenth or eleventh week of fetal development. So it appears that the eggs are available for harvesting at ages when many abortions are performed.

Still, very little is known about the development of eggs in fetuses or about the environment necessary to allow fetal eggs to be fertilized and develop into babies. Despite optimistic assertions to the effect that fetal ovaries may be less vulnerable to rejection by the recipient's natural immunological defense system, a woman who gets a fetal egg or an entire ovary might reject it unless she takes the same battery of immunosuppressive drugs that all organ transplant recipients must now endure. The effects these drugs might have on a pregnancy are not unknown, since women with transplants have had healthy babies, but there are certainly risks involved. The few papers published on the transplantation of adult reproductive organs in animals lend little support to the idea that the transplantation of fetal reproductive organs will prove easy or even possible.

Even less is known about the ability of fetal ovaries to function once they are removed from a body. A woman who wanted fetal eggs might have to be present at the abortion clinic and ready for the transplantation of fetal ovarian tissue as soon as an abortion had been performed. This prospect may in itself be sufficient to dampen any interest in the use of fetal gametes.

Suppose the technical difficulties in fetal ovarian transplants could be overcome. There would still seem to be serious ethical obstacles to allowing this sort of transplantation to be done.

Is it really a good idea to allow sperm, eggs, or embryos to be used without the consent of the person to whom they belong? Should the law allow someone to be born without the permission of the parent from whom an egg or sperm is obtained? At least one state court, the Tennessee Supreme Court in its ruling on the Davis case, a custody dispute over frozen embryos being kept in storage at a fertility clinic, held that it would be against public policy to force persons to become parents against their will (see chapter 1). If parenting without the explicit consent of those whose gametes are used is wrong, then fetuses would obviously be off-limits for harvesting reproductive tissues.

Moreover, would it really be in the best interest of a child to be born from the egg of an aborted fetus? Would women from whose fetuses fetal eggs are procured have the right to claim custody over any child born via transplant should they learn the identity of that child? What would the impact be on a child to learn that its grandmother had aborted its mother but consented to the use of fetal eggs? True, kids adapt to all sorts of circumstances and challenges, but one might hope medicine could come up with a better source of eggs than aborted fetuses.

Fetal egg donation is the latest in a series of stunning promissory notes about how science is changing the way babies are made. Grandmothers have given birth to their own grandchildren, postmenopausal women have had babies, the first tentative steps toward the creation of human embryo clones have been taken, and a technique has been announced for modifying the genetic makeup of cells that create sperm, thereby opening the door to the possibility of germline engineering and eugenics (Brinster, 1995). Science is challenging our definitions of mother, father, parent, and child. Society needs to decide whether morality requires that some of the proposed revisions ought to be rejected. To do so, it must rest its policies and arguments on a clear understanding of the science and technology involved. The controversy over the use of fetal tissue obtained from abortions gives little reason for optimism about the direction future debates might take.

PART TWO

STARTING AND STOPPING MEDICAL TREATMENT FOR THE VERY YOUNG AND VERY OLD

five

Hard Cases Make Bad Law: The Legacy of the Baby Doe Controversy

WELL OVER A DECADE HAS PASSED SINCE the heated controversy flared over the wisdom of the federal government's enacting the so-called Baby Doe regulations for the care of newborns. These regulations, promulgated in March 1983 by the Civil Rights Division of the Department of Health and Human Services, originally required the posting of warning notices in neonatal nurseries concerning the duty to treat handicapped newborns. They also mandated the creation of federal "flying squads" of medical investigators capable of rushing to hospitals where discrimination in treatment had been alleged (DHHS, 1983). These regulations, or, more accurately, a slightly modified version of them issued on January 12, 1984, were eventually held to be unconstitutional by the United States Supreme Court in a 1986 decision, *Bowen vs. American Hospital Association*.

In October 1984, Congress, after lengthy negotiations with provider organizations, professional societies, disability groups, and right-to-life groups, enacted the Child Abuse Amendments of 1984. This law led to federal regulations being issued in April 1985 governing the care of newborns (DHHS, 1985). These regulations require the treatment of all newborns, with only these exceptions: when a newborn infant is chronically and irreversibly comatose, if treatment will merely prolong dying and would not be effective in ameliorating or correcting all of an infant's life-threatening conditions or when the provision of treatment would be virtually futile as well as inhumane. Under all circumstances, nutrition, hydration, and medication are to be provided to infants. State child-protective services are given the responsibility of monitoring and enforcing these regulations.

Assessing the impact of the debate about the Baby Doe regulations and the Child Abuse Amendments of 1984 on infants, their parents, and health care providers is no simple task. Medical care for newborns has hardly remained static in the years since the first Baby Doe regulations were promulgated. Extracorporeal membrane oxygenation, liquid ventilation, and infant heart transplantation are among the many advances that have been introduced into neonatology in the decade since the Baby Doe Law went into effect. Professional and public opinions concerning the medical treatment of newborns, the acceptability of discontinuing medical treatment for any patient, whether adult or child, and the significance of impairment in influencing the quality of life a child or an adult may enjoy have all changed since the passage of the Child Abuse Amendments.

At the time of the controversy over the need for federal regulations, many who were critical of the effort to permit governmental oversight of clinical decision making (Murray and Caplan, 1985; Rhoden, 1986; Caplan, 1984a, 1987a) argued that the Baby Doe regulations were badly thought out and superfluous. The regulations "solved" a problem that was very limited in scope and had no clear-cut right or wrong answer, using rules that were inappropriate, offensively intrusive, and highly insensitive. To call the Baby Doe rules a blunt instrument would be generous. Those who felt federal oversight was appropriate and long overdue argued that the federal government had a legitimate interest in protecting the lives of newborn children and not only should but must intervene to protect their rights (Department of Health and Human Services, 1983; Gerry, 1985; Wilkie, 1991).

The Cases That Triggered the Controversy

Why was there such a disparity of opinion about the treatment of newborn infants in U.S. hospitals? Why did persons concerned about the best interests of children come to such different conclusions about the proper role for government, parents, and third parties with respect to their medical care? And have the laws and regulations that resulted from the Baby Doe controversies had their intended result? To answer these questions it is necessary to understand the kinds of issues and the sorts of value disagreements that divided the parties in the controversy.

The initial national debate about the medical treatment of newborns was triggered by the famous Baby Doe case. A baby born on April 9, 1982, in Bloomington, Indiana, with Down's syndrome and an esophageal atresia died six days later when his parents refused to consent to lifesaving surgery to fix the atresia, or hole, in the esophagus. Without the surgery the child could not eat, and when the parents refused surgery and life support the baby starved to death.

The controversy over the treatment and nontreatment of newborns deepened with the birth of Baby Jane Doe on October 11, 1983, in Long Island, New York. This child was born with spina bifida, hydrocephalus, microcephaly, spasticity, and an apparently malformed brain stem. Her parents, given the option of a surgical intervention to help treat the hydrocephalus or a conservative course of nursing care, chose not to consent to the surgery (Murray and Caplan, 1985). They did, however, consent to artificial life support and palliative care. This baby lived, but the decision to refuse surgery set off a storm of criticism that reached as high as the office of the then newly appointed surgeon general of the United States, C. Everett Koop.

In both cases, third parties tried to make courts intervene in order to assure access to medically efficacious treatment for these infants. In the Baby Doe case, officials from the State of Indiana, in response to a request from a nurse at the hospital where Baby Doe lay dying, were in the process of seeking an order from a federal judge to compel treatment when the newborn died. In the Baby Jane Doe case, the federal government, in response to media reports and legal action by right-to-life groups, attempted to intervene to obtain the medical records of the child in order to ascertain whether treatment would be beneficial. A storm of controversy ensued over the appropriateness of any third-party interventions in cases such as these (Weir, 1984; Murray and Caplan, 1985).

It is interesting that the debate in the United Kingdom over the nontreatment of newborn infants during the early 1980s also focused on cases involving newborns with congenital impairments. In the 1981 case known as "re B (Minor)," the parents of a child with Down's syndrome and duodenal atresia decided not to have surgery performed to correct the atresia, knowing this would mean the death of their baby. Most of the doctors they consulted agreed with their position, but not all did. Eventually legal proceedings commenced which resulted in the baby's being made a ward of the court. The baby was operated upon and placed in foster care.

The other landmark British case involved the decision of a doctor to abide by parental wishes not to provide food or water to a child with Down's syndrome. The pediatrician, Dr. Leonard Arthur, was originally charged with murder and later tried for attempted murder. He was acquitted after a widely publicized and controversial trial (Brahams and Brahams, 1983).

These cases became the paradigms or exemplars that grounded public and professional debate about the treatment of newborns in the English-speaking world.

Does the Federal Government Have a Place at the Bedside?

Some critics of the Baby Doe regulations maintained that there were simply no circumstances that would ever justify intervention by federal officials into the practices of neonatal nurseries. Local and state governments, child-protective services, and local and state courts were seen as entirely adequate to the task of regulating the clinical care given to newborn children. Even simple requests by federal officials to review records and medical histories of particular children were criticized as being unduly intrusive.

The dispute about the proper role of the federal government in ensuring the civil rights of children was fraught with irony. Many who had argued for an aggressive federal role in enforcing civil rights laws with respect to minorities and women—such as the American Civil Liberties Union; professional associations of lawyers, doctors, and nurses; and feminists— maintained that the federal government had no business snooping around neonatal units. Many conservative groups, public officials, and civic organizations who on other issues maintained that the federal government should play a minimal role in the lives of citizens and who touted the glories of local control and individual autonomy in resolving matters of individual behavior, were in the front ranks of the effort to assign an oversight and enforcement role to the federal government with respect to treatment decisions for newborns.

Consider one example. The same Civil Rights Division officials in the Reagan administration who pressed the original Baby Doe regulations in the federal courts also argued, at roughly the same time, that the federal government had no right to impose federal civil rights statutes upon Grove City College. In this case a private school held that it was not accountable to federal affirmative action requirements because it did not accept any direct federal funds to support scholarships or athletic programs. The federal government entered this case on the side of Grove City College, arguing that colleges which accepted federal money to support particular programs were not bound to apply federal civil rights laws governing women and minorities to other programs not directly and explicitly supported by federal funds. The same officials argued that section 504 of the Rehabilitation Act of 1973 did apply to the care of newborns in any U.S. hospital, public or private, on the grounds that hospitals that accepted any federal money, including Medicare and Medicaid payments, were bound by the law in all programs even though the 1973 law made no explicit mention of newborns or medical care.

The disagreement about the need to monitor and regulate the treatment of newborns was in many ways a stalking horse for a more general debate about the proper role of government with respect to clinical autonomy in health care. In fact, much of the resistance on the part of organized medicine, especially the American Medical Association and various state medical societies who weighed in in opposition to the efforts of the administration and some members of Congress to legislate and regulate in the area of the medical care of newborns, was more indicative of general resistance to any government intrusion into the practice of medicine as it was specific opposition to the presence of federal officials in neonatal nurseries or protecting parental rights against government mandates.

While some believe (Nimz, 1989) that the job of protecting the welfare of newborns belongs to the federal government, since state child-protective services have bungled the job or are unwilling to take the job seriously, this view has relatively few adherents. Legally, the monitoring of abuse and neglect has long been a responsibility of the states, not the federal government. Indeed, there is a certain amount of variation permitted to the states with respect to what constitutes neglect or abuse in such areas as religious refusals of treatment.

The reality of newborn care is that there is no way for government to directly monitor or control what happens. A physician, nurse, social worker, or member of the clergy must be willing to report what is going on in the care of the child to an outside authority. Even accrediting organizations in health care must rely upon the good-faith quality control of providers and families in order to know whether the care given by a particular hospital is adequate. Even though the Baby Doe laws remain on the books, the case for transferring oversight responsibility to the federal government or a federal agency has never been made. There are too many births, events move too quickly, and the system is too reliant on the monitoring and whistle-blowing activities of providers and parents to think that any federal agency could directly monitor or intervene.

This does not mean that the federal government and federal agencies ought not have some ability to review cases and retrospectively assess care. It is one thing to allow federal officials outside the clinical setting the right to override provider decisions in the neonatal nursery. It is a different matter to argue that federal agencies ought to have the authority to retrospectively see charts and records to assess the quality of care being provided in neonatal units. The latter function is consistent with the federal government's responsibility to assure that minimal standards of quality medical care are delivered at institutions where the federal government is directly paying for the care of patients, including newborns.

Babies Doe and the Scope of Law and Regulations

Some of the most vehement critics of a federal role in monitoring the care of newborns, such as myself, felt the content of the proposed federal regulations and the revised law that was subsequently enacted were seriously flawed. The paradigmatic cases used in articulating the scope and meaning of the regulations were confusing and atypical (Caplan, 1984a; Murray and Caplan, 1985).

The cases that motivated concern on the part of Surgeon General Koop, the Department of Health and Human Services, and, ultimately, many members of Congress and President Reagan about the adequacy of the care being given to newborn children in neonatal units were cases of children born with Down's syndrome or spina bifida. This focus, while appropriate for those troubled by claims that the infants in the Baby Doe and Baby Jane Doe cases did not receive proper, necessary, and efficacious medical care, created grave problems for the formulation of public policy that still haunt the fields of neonatology and pediatrics.

Treatment practices with respect to spina bifida and Down's syndrome were rapidly changing from what they had been in the 1960s and 1970s. Down's syndrome was once seen as a hopeless condition in which a child would have the capacity for only minimal intellectual functioning. Spina bifida was a condition for which no real treatments existed. As knowledge of Down's syndrome grew, so did medicine's understanding of the range of behavior and intellectual capacity associated with this genetic condition. Surgical and medical techniques for treating spina bifida evolved which permitted fluid to be drained from the brain thereby preventing damage. Clinical practice began to change with respect to treatment and nontreatment decisions. Federal officials, right-to-life groups, and some disability groups were seeking changes in medical practice that were already changing of their own momentum.

What is especially disturbing in terms of the controversy that the Baby

Doe battle represented is that kids with impairments such as Down's syndrome and spina bifida did not represent the range or complexity of treatment decisions that parents and their health care providers faced. Other kinds of anomalies, impairments, and disabilities created by prematurity and prenatal injury were lumped together with questions of when to treat or not treat a baby born with a handicap. The kinds of cases and treatment issues addressed by existing federal law and regulations under the Child Abuse Amendments of 1984 were not in the early 1980s and are certainly not today the cases that raise the hardest moral problems for parents, health care providers, and society.

Current regulations and existing law address the issue of the treatment of newborns under the framework of child abuse and neglect. The original attempt to regulate the treatment of newborns, however, was promoted under a framework of discrimination against the handicapped. The legal foundation upon which the original Baby Doe regulations rested was the prohibition of discrimination against those with disabilities as enjoined by section 504 of the Rehabilitation Act of 1973. The discrimination focus was a result of the fact that much of the concern about the fate of children in neonatal nurseries was exclusively focused on infants born with congenital impairments and disabilities.

The scope of later versions of the regulations and eventually of the Child Abuse Amendments of 1984 expanded to include discussions of when treatment could and could not be withheld from children born very prematurely, with very low birth weight, or with injuries resulting from drugs, abuse, or the process of birth itself. After the Supreme Court invalidated the appropriateness of the discrimination framework, the foundation of the law changed to abuse and neglect (Rhoden and Arras, 1985). The range of cases captured under this framework involves many kinds of treatment decisions for a very diverse set of newborns, some with impairments, some whose only "impairment" was extreme prematurity, and some with impairments so severe that they were incompatible with life regardless of the medical care that might be given. It is simply wrong to equate the treatment decisions that parents and providers face in deciding what to do about the fate of a 450-gram, twenty-two-week-old neonate with the choices that are faced when a baby with Down's syndrome requires surgery to repair a hole in the esophagus. Despite the shift in the philosophical foundation for federal regulation, the change in treatment practices for spina bifida and Down's, and the expansion of the range of cases to be covered, treatment decisions about infants born with Down's or spina bifida dominated and incredibly continue to dominate both political and popular discussions of the appropriateness of legislating medical care by the federal government and treatment decisions that parents make for their babies.

The Impact of Federal Law and Regulation: Have the Baby Doe Regulations Done Any Good?

Relatively few studies have been conducted of the impact of federal laws and regulations or, in some parts of the country, of state laws on the practice of neonatology or the treatment of newborns. The little information that does exist does not support the view that federal intervention was necessary. Nor does it support the position that federal action has been beneficial for infants or their families.

In 1987, the Office of the Inspector General of the Department of Health and Human Services conducted a survey of state child abuse and neglect agencies to determine compliance with the 1984 federal law. The investigation found that in the two years since the Baby Doe regulations had been issued, twenty-two cases of possible abuse or neglect had been reported. State child-protective agencies felt the evidence was such as to merit an investigation in six cases. There were more than three million births in U.S. hospitals during this period. Six cases represent an absurdly tiny percentage of those births. It was not clear to the investigators that state agency intervention had changed the treatment of a newborn in any of the six cases.

Reports of infant abuse or neglect under the child abuse regulations that bind child-protective agencies in many states (a few states have declined federal funds for child abuse and are, as a result, not bound by the regulations) have, if anything, decreased since 1987. The fact that no physician, hospital, or nurse in the United States has been found civilly or criminally liable under the provisions of the 1984 act and 1985 regulations would tend to corroborate the position that the law and regulations now on the books were not merited by a "holocaust" in U.S. neonatal units, which some advocacy groups and editorialists alleged existed. Nor has federal intervention under the framework of child abuse and neglect helped shed much light on the key moral dilemmas which still trouble parents and their providers in caring for neonates.

The few subsequent studies of neonatal practices and provider attitudes that have been done show that some newborns may have received overly aggressive and arguably inappropriate care (Koppelman, Irons, and Koppelman, 1988; Young and Stevenson, 1990). These studies hint that federal law and regulation may be doing more harm than good for infants and their families, either by forcing interventions upon infants that are simply not justified in terms of their efficacy or by allowing some providers to fuzz the line between research and therapy.

Ironically, the major outcome of the Baby Doe regulations seems to be that some infants who are born extremely premature wind up getting full-press, aggressive interventions with less choice being given to their parents. Experimentation and innovation in neonatology have flourished with respect to premature infants. The medical care of children born with mild or moderate congenital impairments seems to have remained stable throughout the late 1980s. There has undoubtedly been much more discussion about the medical care and rights of children with disabilities than there would have been if the Baby Doe controversy had never erupted. But the level and degree of care given to children with spina bifida or Down's today seems to reflect an increased understanding of these conditions by health care providers more than it does federal efforts to prohibit or penalize discrimination.

Paradigmatic Cases and the Meaning of Disability

Recent scholarship in bioethics has emphasized the importance of paradigmatic cases in understanding how moral analysis produces consensus (Caplan, 1989a; Hoffmeister, Freedman, and Fraser, 1989; Moreno, 1995). Nowhere is the role of paradigmatic cases more in evidence than in the Baby Doe controversy. The emergence of the Bloomington Baby Doe and the Long Island Baby Jane Doe cases as defining the scope and content of moral debate for most Americans meant that the focus of this debate was on children whose needs and problems did not and still do not represent the full range of newborn children whose medical problems raise complex ethical questions about starting and stopping treatment (Weir and Bale, 1989; Bay and Burgess, 1991).

The battle over the role government should take in protecting the welfare and health of newborns was fought in the early 1980s on the terrain of disability and handicap, and within that domain only a narrow set of impairments were used as exemplars. The Baby Doe, Baby B (minor), and Baby Jane Doe cases involved decisions by parents not to offer medical treatment to children who were born with congenital impairments. The real question was whether parents had allowed children to die only because they had been born with impairments. There can be no doubt that some infants born with congenital impairments were not treated by doctors in the hope that they would die—and that some of them did die (Duff and Campbell, 1973; Lorber, 1972; Gerry, 1985). It was then and remains now appropriate for third parties to inquire into the medical care given to newborn infants with impairments. Given what was known and what could be done in the way of treatment, the nontreatment of newborns with congenital disabilities such as Down's syndrome or spina bifida was simply immoral by the early 1980s.

One of the most frequently cited articles by those who believed that the "holocaust" in U.S. neonatal units demanded prompt and decisive action by the federal government was a piece in the *New England Journal of Medicine* by Raymond Duff and A. G. M. Campbell. This article reported that 43 of the 299 deaths which occurred in the special care nursery at the Yale–New Haven Hospital from 1970 to 1972 followed decisions to withdraw treatment (Duff and Campbell, 1973). Defenders of the disabled were outraged at this report.

Many infants with spina bifida, Down's syndrome, and other congenital disorders were allowed to die in U.S. and British neonatal nurseries in the 1960s and early 1970s. However, by the early 1980s, the prevention of deaths such as those that occurred in the 1960s and early 1970s had become the standard of care. In the 1960s, interventions such as artificial feeding and fluid provision for newborns either did not exist or were not well understood. Even the efficacy of shunts in the treatment of hydrocephalus remained controversial (Lorber, 1972). This was no longer true by the mid-1980s, when the use of shunts and the management of technology in intensive care units had made great strides.

A major impact of the federal law and regulations that were enacted as a result of the controversy was to affirm the rights, worth, and interests of children born with impairments and congenital birth defects. Perhaps the battle over the Baby Doe laws contributed to the public's and the medical profession's understanding of these conditions. Nonetheless, the fight over the DHHS regulations and continuing disagreements about the impact of and need for subsequent law was greatly complicated by the fact that the parties involved in the debate did not see eye to eye about the urgency of affirming the rights and worth of these newborns. Instead the battle was joined over the issue of who would have authority over medical treatment—parents, doctors, or third parties.

The overwhelming majority of health care professionals were, by the time the controversy erupted, convinced that treatment for infants born with congenital anomalies made sense. Those in the disability and right-to-life movements were not convinced that the interests of these children would be adequately protected by health care providers and families who might still have strong biases against disability (Asch and Fine, 1988; Gerry, 1985). Sadly, in terms of the energy and anger wasted on the Baby Doe debate, the locus of moral uncertainty had shifted by the time the debate began.

Health care professionals involved in the care of newborns were much more troubled at the time the Baby Doe debate erupted about the treatment of newborns who were born extremely premature or with severe illnesses or injuries. They felt the Baby Doe laws and regulations were of little help in that they applied standards appropriate for one category of newborn, those with congenital impairment, to other children whose medical problems were of an entirely different and much less well understood nature (Bay and Burgess, 1991). The fact that the wrong babies were the paradigmatic cases made the analysis of moral problems in the neonatal nursery much more difficult and much more frustrating for parents and health care providers dealing with these children.

Part of the problem with focusing only upon cases of spina bifida and Down's as paradigmatic is that other sorts of disabilities, far more severe and devastating, were equated with these. For example, children born with anencephaly can be and have been described as disabled. It would seem more accurate to describe a child with most of its brain missing, unable to think or feel or sense, as unabled. Similarly, to call children with Lesch-Nyhan's syndrome or Tay-Sachs disabled is to distort the meaning of disability beyond recognition.

On the other hand, focusing on only certain forms of disability obscures the fact that many children born in neonatal units are not disabled but at risk of death due to prematurity. A child born at 450 grams is not accurately described as disabled. That infant may or may not develop disabilities. To say that medical treatment must be given to a 450-gram neonate on the grounds that anything less would constitute abuse or neglect is simply to fail to understand the difference between disability and prematurity and between experimentation and treatment. No one knows what will happen if treatment is given to babies born extremely prematurely. When outcomes are unknown and highly uncertain, it is conceptually muddled to equate the treatment of babies born premature with those born with impairments and handicaps. But that is precisely what the Baby Doe rule did when it was first promulgated, and that is a confusion that continues to stalk the field of neonatology to the present day.

Do Parents Care about Their Kids?

In the time I have spent in neonatal nurseries, nothing has impressed me more than the love nearly all parents have for their child and their almost compulsive desire to do what is best for it. No matter how sick, how impaired, or how different their child might be, with very few exceptions the parents I have encountered have quickly bonded to their newborn baby and have sought only the best of care for their child. This bond between parent and child has been reported by many others with far more experience than mine. Nurses, doctors, parents, and social scientists who have spent time around newborn nurseries are impressed with the level of parental caring that exists despite the technology and the often uncertain prognosis (Frohock, 1986; Guillemin and Holmstrom, 1987; Anspach, 1993). There certainly are parents who would abandon or even injure a child whom they perceived to be less than perfect or burdensome (Asch and Fine, 1988; Murray and Caplan, 1985; Powell and Hecimovic, 1985; Anspach, 1993), but such parents are in the minority.

There is no reason to think that parents in the early 1970s were any less likely to bond to and love their babies than they were in the 1980s or are today. What is different is that in the 1960s and 1970s, Down's syndrome and spina bifida were both considered conditions that would inevitably lead to lives of misery (Crocker and Cullinane, 1972; Lorber, 1972). Parents were told that no cures were possible, that severe retardation and disability were certain, and that the ultimate and sole destination for most children with Down's syndrome or spina bifida would be state-run institutions or asylums—institutions that parents often believed to be under-funded and horrible. With this kind of bleak prognosis, it is not surprising that many parents would elect nontreatment for their children. To many parents, it must have seemed kinder to allow their child to die than to face a life of misery (Powell and Hecimovic, 1985). A decision for nontreatment made during this time cannot be equated with indifference or hostility to the child, as those who refuse medical treatment for their children on religious grounds such as Jehovah's Witnesses or Christian Scientists correctly point out.

In the two decades that have elapsed since the publication of Duff and Campbell's landmark paper and the publication of Lorber about his experience in deciding whether or not to treat newborns with spina bifida in his nursery, much has changed in what is known about and the ability to do something positive about the medical problems associated with congenital anomalies. Experts now know, having been pushed to look by disability groups and parent associations, that Down's syndrome refers to a range of potential outcomes, not a single, stereotypic presentation. The same is true for spina bifida.

Looking through the retrospectoscope, it is difficult to understand a decision to allow a child born with spina bifida to remain unshunted and untreated. Yet medical opinion concerning spina bifida and Down's was so dire in the 1960s and 1970s that recommendations not to treat were commonplace.

One of the first cases presented to me when I was starting to teach bioethics at Columbia University's Medical Center was that of a newborn infant, Ellen, who had been born with spina bifida and a variety of other anomalies. Her doctors were convinced that the lesion was so high on the spinal cord that the baby would always be paralyzed from the waist down and incontinent of both bowel and bladder. They also felt the degree of hydrocephalus already present had so damaged the baby's brain that she would be permanently and severely retarded. They advised the family against any treatment, including the placement of a shunt. A number of them told me that they hoped Ellen would succumb to an infection, since her prognosis was grim indeed. I was persuaded by their predictions of a life of utter suffering and misery that the right thing to do was not to treat Ellen.

Ellen's parents were not. The family refused to listen to these grim forecasts about their daughter. They had no previous children, and Ellen was very much a wanted child. They insisted she be shunted. They took her home and gave her meticulous nursing care. The father later spent much of his time building toys and special transportation equipment for his paralyzed daughter.

My last contact with Ellen came when she was eight. She had grown into a vivacious, charming, happy, and outgoing kid. She was paralyzed from the waist down and confined to a wheelchair. She was incontinent. And she required constant help in feeding, bathing, toileting, and other activities of daily living. But Ellen was certainly much loved and giving a lot of love back to her parents. The mere thought that she might have been allowed to die filled them with nothing but dread. The fact that I had concurred with those who had said eight years earlier that she would be better off dead left me with the same feeling.

Today, many argue that Baby Jane Doe might have gone on to live a life like Ellen's if her parents had been cajoled or forced into having her shunted sooner than they did by the intervention of the federal government (Andrusko, 1991; Koop, 1991; Wilkie, 1991). And they may be correct. Hindsight does show that at least some infants proved their doctors wrong. The fact that children like Ellen flourished does not mean that the physicians and nurses who believed that the prognosis for infants with spina bifida or Down's syndrome was very grim were not acting in good faith, or even that they were wrong. It does show that medical decision making sometimes must proceed with a high degree of uncertainty and that different parents and doctors may respond differently in the face of uncertainty (Rhoden, 1986; Caplan, 1987a).

From a public policy standpoint, Ellen and Baby Jane Doe raise the obvious question of whether it was right fifteen years ago or is right today to attempt to legislate a single standard of care in response to uncertainty about prognosis or outcome in the care of children. While kids like Ellen show the terrible price of making a wrong choice and failing to treat, I remain unconvinced that government can do a better job than parents in deciding what is best for babies.

Public policy must presume that parents love their children, seek what is best for them, and will act accordingly. The burden should be on others, be they providers or government officials, to show that these presumptions are false. That is not the spirit which motivated the original Baby Doe regulations and, unfortunately, it is not always the spirit which guides their application in the neonatal and pediatric intensive care units of today.

Government has a duty to watch out for the interests of children. In carrying out this duty, government must tread very carefully in the hospital. The cases that command the greatest public attention and concern may not be those that raise the hardest moral questions, as the Baby Doe debate amply demonstrates. The only practical way regulation with respect to decisions about starting and stopping medical care for children can be effective is by trying to work with parents and health care providers rather than simply pushing them away from the bedside.

six

Analogies to the Holocaust and Contemporary Bioethical Disputes about Assisted Suicide and Euthanasia

ONE OF THE MOST COMMON ARGUMENTS invoked in bioethics today is what might be termed the Nazi analogy. I will use this shorthand phrase to describe comparisons that make essential reference to the Holocaust, to the conduct of Nazis, or to experiments, public health measures, or euthanasia programs carried out by German doctors and scientists before and during the Second World War. The Nazi analogy is invoked by those who believe that these historical events have a moral equivalent or parallel in contemporary conduct or policy.

The Nazi analogy is quite powerful. It is arguably the most serious charge that can be made in bioethics. Yet contemporary bioethics has chosen to ignore this most powerful of claims. And that is unfortunate given the frequency with which the analogy appears in current discussions and controversies.

For many years, I wrote a weekly syndicated newspaper column about ethical issues in medicine and science. Among the letters and e-mail messages I received, many began by saying, "Don't you know what the Nazis did?" If a reader was especially infuriated by some argument or claim I made, they sometimes said, "You are a Nazi."

This sort of glib invocation of the Nazi analogy is not limited to those moved to write letters to columnists. It is not all that rare at an academic conference to hear a speaker invoke the Holocaust or mention the conduct of the Nazis in debates about euthanasia, gene therapy, abortion, or the use of fetal tissue for transplant research. The Nazi analogy may be less common in academic writings than in letters to the editor, but probably only slightly.

A few years ago, Peter Singer, a philosopher from Monash University in Australia, went to Germany, where various universities had invited him to give some talks. He was to speak, among other things, about his views concerning the termination of treatment for newborn babies in intensive care settings. Singer has written many articles and books in support of the view that some newborns ought to be allowed to die without any effort being made to treat their ailments or dysfunctions.

Singer's controversial views about the nontreatment of severely and hopelessly ill newborns are well known. He has written and lectured extensively about his view that in some cases severely disabled infants should be allowed to die if that is what their parents desire. The universities who had invited him had to have known about his views. Some within the German disability and environmental movements certainly did. And they did not want to hear them.

Demonstrators, including some with disabilities, came to his lectures to protest and shout him down. They argued vociferously that he should not be allowed to speak because he was echoing arguments that the Nazis had made. Many accused Singer of actually being a Nazi. Singer's views were condemned as similar to those held by the persons responsible for the Holocaust.

Singer found these attacks personally devastating. Here he was, a Jew from Australia who had come to Germany, being picketed, shouted down, and attacked as a Nazi. The criticism worked. Singer's lecture tour came to an abrupt halt.

Of course, the mere fact that individuals are Jewish does not mean they are incapable of espousing Nazi-like views. Singer, however, felt the Nazi analogy was completely inappropriate as a response to his views about the treatment and nontreatment of disabled newborns. Was he right? Were those who passionately opposed his views too quick or glib or simply irresponsible in invoking the Nazi analogy?

In 1993, when I directed the University of Minnesota's Center for Biomedical Ethics, the center sponsored a conference that focused on termination of treatment issues which a number of families had faced with dying loved ones. Among those who spoke were family members who had been involved in many of the most widely known right-to-die cases: Cruzan, Busalacchi, Quinlan, Delio, Wanglie, and Brophy. Protesters who opposed euthanasia tried to disrupt the conference. They invoked the Nazi analogy loudly and insistently.

Joe Cruzan, the father of Nancy Cruzan, whose food and water were disconnected after a long court fight that went all the way up to the United States Supreme Court, was one of the speakers. His daughter had died in 1991 just after Christmas. Joe, who five years later took his own life, recalled in his talk the great anger he had felt when he and his wife went to the nursing home to say goodbye to Nancy, or Nan as he called her. He could not believe that not only did he have to deal with the emotions associated with allowing his daughter to die, but he also had to put up with cries of "Nazis" being screamed at them as they came and went. Even as he spoke at the Minnesota conference, protesters were busy distributing literature invoking the Nazi analogy outside in the lobby of the conference hotel. Joe Cruzan knew firsthand the power and force of the Nazi analogy—it can really hurt.

The Nazi analogy is not confined to the street or picket signs. The analogy appears often in books and learned journals. Typical of such invocations which can be found through a cursory search of editorials, letters to the editor, articles, books, and reviews are "abortion is America's Holocaust," "Dr. Kevorkian will lead us, if unchecked, down the path to Dachau and Auschwitz," "the Germans started with the retarded and then moved to the senile and then . . ." (Caplan, 1992c).

Such analogies or arguments are general invocations of the Nazi analogy—they make no specific reference to events, policies, or actions. They use the Holocaust in a generic way. The version of the analogy holds that general comparison between then and now is appropriate and telling.

The analogy can and does take more precise forms. For instance, some contend that germline genetic engineering is immoral because of its relationship to and precedent in the application of race hygiene in the Nazi regime to marriage laws. In the debate over the use of fetal tissue from elective abortions for transplantation research, analogies were often made between this research and the use of data from Nazi medical experiments conducted in concentration camps (see chapter 4). That analogy appears, for example, in the minority report of a special committee convened by an assistant secretary of the Department of Health and

Human Services, James Mason, to examine the issue. The advisory committee voted not to ban the federal funding of such research or prohibit it, but the Bush administration maintained a ban partly on the basis of this sort of moral objection (Vawter and Caplan, 1992).

Another example of what might be called the specific or focused use of the Nazi analogy arose with reference to the Baby Doe controversy (see chapter 5) and, more recently, the case of Baby K. Baby K is a child who spent much of her life in an intensive care unit in a hospital in Virginia. The child was born with most of its brain missing. She was not capable of thought or mental activity. Nonetheless, the child's mother insisted that all efforts to keep the baby alive be undertaken and that when the baby's heart or breathing stopped that she be resuscitated.

The hospital went to federal court to obtain permission to stop life-sustaining care. Some critics of that action argued that stopping care would be morally akin to the secret euthanasia program undertaken at Hitler's orders in 1939 to eliminate children with disabilities. Opinion pieces in newspapers such as *USA Today* argued that to allow Baby K to die despite the mother's wishes would be doing precisely to the child what the Nazis had done to disabled children in the T2 euthanasia program in Germany just before the start of the war.

Another invocation of the focused or specific form of the Nazi analogy often appears in radical animal-rights literature. Demonstrators shout and pamphlets contend that experimentation on animals now being conducted in U.S. research facilities will someday be seen as akin to the experimentation done on concentration camp inmates.

The Nazi analogy can also arise when comparing instances of immoral conduct in one time period to those in another. I spoke at a conference at Brandeis University, located just outside of Boston, in 1993 to discuss the notorious Tuskegee study in which African American men were left untreated by public health service doctors even though the doctors knew that they had syphilis and that a cure existed (see chapter 2). One person from the audience was very upset by my presentation of the Tuskegee story. She said that the Tuskegee experiment is "just like what happened to us," meaning "the Jews," in the concentration camps. Some people came up to me after my remarks and complained that they felt that some of the African American panelists who appeared on the program with me were too adamant in saying that the Tuskegee study was unique. The position of these audience members was that the Nazi analogy, used in a focused way, is sometimes legitimate and appropriate. Blacks and Jews have something in common. They both suffered abuses in the name of science or at the hands of scientists. Why insist on differences when in fact there are parallels between what took place in the experiments done in the concentration camps and the Tuskegee study?

These examples are only a small fraction of the many Nazi analogies made in contemporary bioethical debates. They suffice to show that the analogy comes in two forms—general and specific. And these examples also suffice to show that the Nazi analogy is one of the most powerful arguments that exists in bioethical discourse. If you can persuasively invoke the Nazi analogy, it is taken for granted that you will win the moral argument. If you can make this charge stick, it has sufficient moral force to show that your opponent's position is simply not credible.

Arguments by analogy of this power deserve more comment than those in bioethics have given to them, for the Nazi analogy is not used with anything like the care and precision that it deserves. Persons picketing outside Nancy Cruzan's nursing home room, those writing letters to the editor about abortion or genetic engineering, and pundits or TV talk show hosts who heat up the airwaves by drawing facile analogies between the Holocaust and revelations about radiation experiments with retarded children in the United States in the 1950s do so with little thought about the legitimacy or the real power of the analogy. The same can be said about the use of the analogy in the scholarly literature which draws parallels between the use of fetal tissue in research and the use of data from hypothermia experiments at Dachau or experiments on mice and rats and experiments on women at Ravensbruck.

Part of the reason for the widespread appropriation of the Holocaust through the indiscriminate invocation of the Nazi analogy is the relative silence that until recently pervaded the field of bioethics when it came to reflecting on the Holocaust and the role which Nazi medicine and biomedical science played in it (Annas and Grodin, 1992; Caplan, 1992c; and see chapter 2). It is only in the past few years that analyses have started to appear of the ethical issues raised by the brutal experiments in the camps and the creation of a genetically grounded euthanasia program. It is only in the past ten years that scholars such as Bruno Müller-Hill, Robert Proctor, Michael Kater, and Bill Seidelman have begun to do the historical work necessary to help understand the role played by scientists, public health officials, nurses, and physicians in the Holocaust. Even with the emergence of this recent scholarship, too little attention is paid to the questions of what Nazi doctors did, what the ethical rationales for concentration camp experiments were, and what reasons and justifications people gave for their conduct (Caplan, 1992c). The actions of Nazi doctors and researchers remains relatively unexamined terrain.

The scholarly examination of the Nazi analogy is equally unexplored intellectual terrain. There are very few articles on the subject in the literature of bioethics.

Why is that so? Fear about the risks of discussing Nazi ethics is one reason. There is always a danger that the mere presentation of the ethical rationales used by the Nazis for their conduct and policies confers legitimacy upon their horrible acts and terrible deeds.

There is also an aversion to taking a long hard look at what health professionals and scientists did during the years before and throughout the Holocaust. Medicine and science played such a prominent role in the Holocaust that it is hard for those who admire medicine and science to accept. In the decades since the Second World War, there have been many instances of large-scale mass murder in places such as East Timor, Iraq, Somalia, Rwanda, Afghanistan, Bosnia, and Cambodia. Many of these more recent slaughters have their roots in racism. What took place in Germany, however, not only had its roots in racism but a racism that found willing support from mainstream biomedicine. The consequences of that racism were implemented using scientific and engineering technology administered by doctors and healers.

In building a gas chamber, running a transportation network, or selecting who would die based upon a psychological, physical, or anthropological examination, scientists helped engineer the Holocaust. For those who see medicine and science as bound by a higher moral code, that is a very difficult fact to accept.

Still another reason to have steered away from a close examination of the Nazi analogy is uncertainty about how to respond to it. For many years, I didn't know what to say when I heard the analogy made, because I was not sure whether it was valid or not. If someone said that allowing the withdrawal of food, antibiotics, or dialysis from a permanently comatose person is the first step on the road to what took place in Nazi Germany, I did not know enough about history to know what to reply. Nearly every other person in bioethics faced the exact same problem. It is still true today. Part of the reason for silence is that ignorance of history allows the analogy to go unchallenged and unendorsed.

In one sense all analogies are suspect, because an analogy is by definition a comparison between things that are dissimilar in at least some respects. More important, many survivors and students of the Holocaust maintain that the Holocaust is unique, that the sufferings and experiences cannot even be described, much less used as objects of comparison.

Of course, even if one grants the uniqueness of the Holocaust, even the impossibility of accurately describing it, that does not place it beyond comparison. The magnitude of the horror of what took place may be beyond literary, cinematic, or artistic depiction. This might only mean, however, that great care and caution have to be used in making analogies. If the Holocaust is truly beyond adequate description, then what I have termed global or sweeping analogies may be by definition invalid. Those who invoke the Nazi analogy in a broad or general fashion are pressing the limits of valid analogy simply because the broader the scope of their reference, the harder it becomes to understand exactly what they think the Holocaust was and thus why it is of moral relevance to a current issue.

If, however, the analogy is made in a more specific way, to a specific set of events such as the hypothermia experiments or to the T2 euthanasia program for demented elderly persons, then analogies might be possible and plausible. If so, what sorts of standards should be brought to bear to analyze these limited, more focused claims?

To answer this we need to know how people make analogies in other areas. By understanding what constitutes a valid analogy in other domains of life, it may be possible to learn what ought to be expected to defend or justify the invocation of the Nazi analogy in bioethics.

Much has been written on the uses of metaphor, simile, and analogy in literature. But analogy, metaphor, and simile are not the same in poetry, drama, and theater as they are in ethics. I think comparisons or analogies in the arts are meant to provoke, sometimes to puzzle. In other words, the arts use analogies to try to get people to recognize and think about comparisons and similarities that they might not otherwise have noticed.

Analogy does not often play this role in ethics. It's more akin to analogy as used in science. There, comparison is used as an aid to exposition, as a heuristic, as a way to make you think about how to solve a problem in a way that you might not unless you've got an analogy that you can, so to speak, get your mind around. And sometimes analogy is used straight out as a way to explain something. Analogies, as Thomas Kuhn and others have argued, are used in science to ground paradigmatic problems that otherwise might be too abstract or unfamiliar. One place where this form of analogy abounds is in organismic biology.

Those who pursue the study of organisms in nature quickly learn of the importance of classification. In order to come up with generalizations or explanations for the natural world, scientists need to order their findings into categories so that others know what they are referring to. However, there is much dispute in biology about how best to classify animals and plants.

It is a commonly understood fact that many creatures have wings. Bats, birds, and flies all do. Even though the musculature and bone structure of each of these types of creatures may differ, scientists say they all possess wings because the things hanging off all their bodies let the creatures fly through the air.

Now consider the hoof of a horse and of a zebra. They both, to remind any reader who has not looked at a zebra hoof lately, have nails at the end, kind of like our fingernails. They clearly have this hard substance on the end of their toe to provide traction and a buffer. The hoof of the zebra is a lot like the hoof of a horse. The wings of a fly, a bat, and a bird are also similar, because they all allow flight.

But biologists know that similarity in appearance is not always the result of common causes. Some traits or behaviors are similar because they perform the same function and thus have similar properties. The fly wing, the bat wing, and the bird wing have some resemblance, not because of anything internal to the hereditary makeup of these animals but because they all have to get through the air. Only certain shapes, as aeronautical engineers know, will get objects up into and through the air. In fact, some of the same physical requirements are present to move through water and other fluids, which is why a fish's fins, a whale's fins, and a submarine's fins are analogous to each other as well as to the wings of bats and birds. Biologists know that bird, fly, and bat wings are analogous, that there are real similarities between them. But the reason for their similarity is the demands made by the environment.

That is not true about the hoofs of the zebra and the horse. They are analogous but not because of external environmental pressures but because these animals are close biological relatives. Biologists call similarities due to common genetic ancestry homologies. Zebras and horses look like one another, just as do dogs and wolves, as a result of their common genetic makeup.

The biological understanding of similarity reveals something of importance about the Nazi analogy. When biologists make comparisons, they must first try to identify what is similar and what is different between organisms. The first step in any comparison is to closely examine the properties and traits to see if they truly are similar. The first task in making a comparison, in invoking an analogy, is to see what real similarities exist as opposed to what just appear on the surface to be similarities but, under closer inspection, are not.

The next step in making a comparison or analogy is to find out what factors are responsible for producing similarity. Some similarities, as the biological examples show, are accidental; they occur because a common external force causes creatures to resemble one another. Some are merely due to chance, as when both I and my dog are covered in mud because we have both fallen into a bog. Other similarities are rooted in genetics. Creatures resemble one another because they have a common parent or are biological relatives.

Those who wish to use the Nazi analogy in bioethics must identify exactly what it is that is similar between Nazi practice and the contemporary practice they condemn. This means that it is most unlikely that any global invocations of the Holocaust will be valid. If there is real similarity between events from the past and today, an important question still remains if the analogy is to hold—why? Are things similar by chance or because of common causes? If analogies are made without this sort of care, then there is a real risk of error in confusing what biologists would call homology with analogy, of confusing traits that are similar but whose similarities are not the result of common or similar causes.

When I was a little boy, I used to visit a place called the Old Man in the Mountains in New Hampshire. This is a rock formation that looks like a face. I always wondered how God had made this sculpture. Later I learned that wind did it. Men can sculpt figures like this, too, but it would be a grave error to presume that the Old Man in the Mountains is a sculpture because it resembles statues artists have made.

If you listen to or watch the talk shows on radio or television or scan the supermarket tabloids, you know they often present people who discuss evidence that UFOs are visiting Earth. Especially popular bits of evidence are the huge outlines of animals and other objects found high in the mountains of South America. What else, various experts ask, could these huge figures be but landmarks for UFO fleets? Other people, who tend not to get the same type of exposure, suggest that these outlines are pictures done by people of ancient cultures for religious or symbolic reasons having nothing to do with alien spacecraft.

The Old Man in the Mountains, the paintings on the high deserts of South America, and the similarities of bat, bird, and fly wings are all examples where caution is in order if false similarities, analogies, and homologies are to be avoided. The same is true of the Nazi analogy.

Surely the moral weight of the events of the Holocaust requires care when invoking these experiences in moral disputes. Those who do so must be prepared to say precisely which properties or events they think have parallels in the events of today. Whoever invokes the analogy must be prepared to state how what took place in the concentration camp at Dachau, in the construction of the specimen museum of Bolshevik Kommisar Jews, or in the race-mixing laws prohibiting interracial sexual contact enacted during the early years of the Third Reich is analogous to some current event.

Those who are too quick and too facile in involving the Nazi analogy, who hold up a sign saying, "You are a Nazi," whenever someone holds a view or takes a course of action they believe to be evil risk not only being wrong but also demeaning the significance of the Holocaust. It is disrespectful and cheapens the horror of the Holocaust not to understand that care and caution are obligatory where the invocation of this most powerful of analogies is concerned. Even if one rejects the view that the Holocaust is unique or the magnitude of evil involved so great as to be beyond description, there is a need for common sense and caution to prevail in referring to these events in moral argument. Those who see analogies must be specific about what they believe is similar between now and then. Blanket invocations such as "abortion is today's Holocaust" or "legalized euthanasia will lead to Nazi Germany" are to be avoided unless they can truly be supported in the scope of the claim being made. To do otherwise risks making the analogy stand only by taking all of the moral force out of it.

It is not enough to show similarities to make a comparison stand. More work remains if an analogy is to be used correctly. Is the Old Man in the Mountains up there because the wind made him or is he there because somebody went up and chiseled him out, like the presidents at Mount Rushmore? Does the wing of the bat resemble the wing of the bird because the wings have some genetic similarity, because they're responding to some environmental functional demand, or is the resemblance just an accident? Things can appear similar because of many different reasons. Showing that the Nazis permitted and encouraged euthanasia or that forced sterilization was practiced on many camp inmates does not in itself show that there is any real or true similarity between these events and euthanasia or sterilization today.

If specificity and detail are crucial to the valid use of the Nazi analogy, then do we know enough to know when the analogy is false? Are there sufficient details available about particular instances of Nazi conduct so that it is certain that a closer inspection of not only the similarities but also their causes will confirm the analogy's validity?

One area in which the Nazi analogy abounds, as has already been noted, is the termination of treatment. The Nancy Cruzan case involved issues of stopping or forgoing life-saving medical care, including the provision of food and water. Many critics of the actions taken in this and similar cases note that, to paraphrase, people were starved to death in

Nazi Germany, were killed by the state as unworthy of life, and the inmates of mental asylums were often not fed and allowed to die owing to their disabilities. They see a direct parallel with Cruzan's case and thousands of other cases in which food and water are stopped in today's nursing homes and intensive care units. They are wrong, terribly, irresponsibly wrong.

It is true that German doctors allowed elderly demented patients and the mentally ill to die for want of rations. People were in fact denied food when supplies got short. This form of social triage took place in Germany in the First World War as well as the Second World War. The fact that these events took place, however, and that they involved doctors not feeding those in their care, doesn't prove that it is valid to draw an analogy to the decision of the Cruzan family to take a feeding tube away from their daughter and sister.

The overriding rationale for allowing people to die of starvation in Germany prior to the Second World War was discrimination against the mentally ill and retarded. The primary reason for medically supervised starvation during the war was racism. The decision was not to supply food to those who otherwise could have, and certainly would have, eaten it (Caplan, 1992c).

Joe Cruzan did not allow his daughter to starve to death because he thought she was an inferior biological being, a genetic threat to the health of his nation, or because he despised the mentally retarded. He never viewed her as a threat to the public health or even to the public purse. None of these issues drove him to want to relieve his daughter of the burden of artificial life support.

Nancy Cruzan, unlike the residents of German homes for the mentally ill and those in concentration camps, could not eat or drink without technological assistance. If she could have eaten, her parents would have insisted that she be fed. The decision to remove her tube was not made in response to a government directive.

The similarities between the Cruzan case and Nazi policies of mandatory starvation of insane persons or imprisoned Jews, Gypsies, and others do not exist. The Nazi analogy as cited with respect to the termination of treatment is not only false but offensive. It obscures the motives and rationales for what took place in German concentrations camps, nursing homes, and mental asylums (Annas and Grodin, 1992).

This is not to say the analogy is always false or invalid. When people warn against using formulas to determine the fiscal burdensomeness on the state of people or groups as a criterion for rationing health care because they see analogies between such arguments and claims in the writings of some proto-Nazis in the 1920s and 1930s, there may be parallels that are real (Caplan, 1992c). However, most who invoke the Nazi analogy fail to do so within even a minimum of precision. The events of the Holocaust deserve to be treated as more than a hunting ground for political rhetoric. Calling feminists "femi-Nazis" or doctors who perform abortions "Nazis" reveals a callous disregard for the millions who died and suffered at the hands of the Nazi regime. To use the Nazi analogy with abandon is to abandon history.

with care, attentiveness, spiritual support, and conversation than they are undergoing Herculean efforts to secure additional hours or days of life of exceedingly poor quality.

An essential element for hospice to function is trust. There must be trust between the patient and the care provider, the patient and the hospice organization, and the care provider and the patient's family or significant others. Without trust, those seeking hospice services could not be sure that they had really pursued all reasonable courses of medical intervention to extend their lives. They could not be sure that they had not been sent to a hospice to die cheaply rather than to die well. Without trust, the ministrations that are the core of hospice care are neither credible nor, if recent work on the importance of trust to therapeutic efficacy (Mechanic, 1996) is accepted, effective. And without trust, some patients and their families would wonder whether the actions taken by hospice workers were always in the best interest of patients.

Prior to the emergence of the movement to legitimize assisted suicide and euthanasia, those who went to a hospice or used one in their home could place complete trust in their hospice care providers. There was almost no reason to fear that anyone had been placed in hospice prematurely, that someone would be sent to a hospice if there were still potentially efficacious therapies to be tried, or that those providing care would not do everything in their power to extend life while maintaining the dignity and quality of that life. The ethos of hospice, at least the public, overt ethos, was clear and consoling—hastening death, hurrying death, assisting in death had no place in hospice treatment.

Events have changed. One state, Oregon, has enacted a law allowing assisted suicide and others may do so soon. Some high federal courts believe a right to assistance in dying can be found in the U.S. Constitution (*Compassion in Dying v. Washington*, 1996; *Quill v. Vacco*, 1996). Doctors and nurses indicate that they will and should sometimes intentionally bring about the death of a patient, sometimes without the consent of the patient (Cassel and Meier, 1990; Quill, 1993; Asch, 1996). Agree or not, like it or not, these shifts in public policy cast a pall over the historical ethos of hospice and thus over the requisite trust. When hastening death becomes an option, the trust necessary to make hospice function as a place where dying is an unhurried, humane affair is in jeopardy.

With the enactment by popular referendum of a state law in Oregon permitting physicians to prescribe lethal doses on request to those who are terminally ill, the bizarre vindication and quasi-martyrdom of Dr. Jack Kevorkian (Caplan, 1996d), and the controversial and momentous holding by two federal appellate courts that the constitutional protections of liberty, privacy, and equal protection establish the right of competent persons to assistance in suicide and prohibit states from enacting laws to the contrary, hospice's historic abhorrence of suicide is not tenable. The negative liberty to refuse medical treatment is rapidly being joined with the positive right to an entitlement to help in dying in U.S. law. The winds of autonomy are blowing death away from hospice toward a very different location.

Why the Need for Assistance in Dying?

The debate about assisted suicide is always cast in terms of personal self-determination, but it actually has less to do with this value than might be supposed. Individuals have always had the right to end their lives regardless of what others may think of the morality of such an action, and only a handful of the terminally ill are so frail and incompetent that they cannot do so if they so choose. The struggle to legalize assisted suicide is really about a number of other matters: fear, guilt, cost, and dignity. Hospice emerged as one way to respond to these concerns. Assisted suicide is now emerging as another. The two are unlikely to coexist for long.

Fear, not self-determination, is fueling the push toward making assisted suicide by doctors legal. Many people are afraid of being kept alive under circumstances they abhor. But they are also afraid they will lack the means, the knowledge, or even the courage to kill themselves. This means that they want competent help available to them when they die, not because they lack the ability to act freely and autonomously to kill themselves but because they fear they will lack the will power or ability to do what they want to do when the time to do it comes. A lack of courage, the desire not to offend relatives and partners, and the worry that competency may flag at the crucial hour all fuel the fear that makes many Americans favor some form of legalization of assisted suicide (Blendon, 1992).

When fear is mixed with guilt, an especially potent power is created, a power strong enough to undercut support for hospice and elevate assisted suicide to the forefront of public policy. In many circles it is still seen as immoral or sinful to take your own life. Suicide may not be illegal, but many believe it to be immoral. Some are not so sure but do not want to take a chance in the hereafter about the morality of suicide.

Physician assistance in dying relieves the individual of carrying the personal moral burden for ending one's own life. It also spares the individual from having to ask family or friends to carry out this deed. In a society that is eager to assign responsibility for many unpleasant or uncomfortable things to others, especially to professionals, assisted suicide looks like a far more attractive option than taking personal responsibility for the decision to end one's life and then acting upon it.

Cost is also fueling the effort to change the law to allow assistance in dying by doctors. Money is not a welcome visitor at debates about assisted suicide, but it is present nonetheless. Many Americans do not want to spend their resources on the final weeks and days of their dying. Still others believe that it is irresponsible to family and even to society to linger around consuming resources once death is inevitable. And still others believe that the only way this nation is going to solve the fiscal burden of an aging society is to find ways to spend less money on them (Callahan, 1993). While these views are not always bluntly articulated when the discussion turns to care for the dying, they are omnipresent whenever economists and public officials talk behind closed doors. The desire to save money creates an atmosphere in which assisted suicide by physicians looks very attractive, surely more attractive than spending the money it would take to upgrade a flagging long-term and chronic care system and perhaps even more attractive than the smaller amounts of money it would take to provide good-quality hospice services to all who might benefit.

Quality of life, not the quality of one's dying, also is a key ingredient in the assisted suicide debate. Much has been made in the debate over assisted suicide of the importance of controlling pain. And it is true that too many Americans die in pain. However, pain is not the issue which is behind the public interest in assisted suicide. What most Americans fear is the loss of capacities to think and feel, to ambulate and emote, to control their bowels and bladder. They understand that there is every reason to believe that they can be kept comfortable and pain free if they receive even minimally competent medical treatment while dying. But that is not enough.

Severe disability, loss of cognitive function, loss of self-esteem, frailness, and dependency are what people have in mind to avoid if they can choose physician-assisted suicide. Hospice does nothing to answer these quality-of-life concerns, since they have little to do with pain and terminal illness. Assisted suicide has everything to do with them.

For Many, Suffering Is the Issue

Arguments about assisted suicide, especially in the context of hospice as an alternative, often pivot around the issue of how well pain can be controlled in someone with cancer or AIDS. But, in fact, there is nothing to debate. Medicine and nursing know full well how to control most forms of pain. They may fail to do so, but the failure has nothing to do with a lack of general knowledge about pain control. It has to do with inadequate training, callous indifference to patient requests for relief, and culpable stupidity about addiction. Even when aggressive pain relief means risking inadvertent death, most hospice workers are comfortable making pain relief a priority come what may in the form of death as a side-effect. But pain is not the issue when it comes to assisted suicide.

The real issue for many who favor assisted suicide is that it provides a way out of a future that some do not wish to endure. If you suffer from a massive stroke, Alzheimer's disease, severe multiple sclerosis, massive burns, a paralyzing injury, ALS, or Parkinsonism, you are not terminally ill. You may not even be in pain. But you most assuredly could find yourself suffering, either anticipating or enduring these dread afflictions.

The moral challenge medicine and nursing face is what to do about the management of suffering, not pain. Suffering is far broader than pain. Suffering refers to the loss of identity that occurs with a disfiguring or disabling injury. Suffering connotes the state of affairs that exists when you know you can no longer remember your children's names or where you live. Suffering is represented by the reality of being made a prisoner inside your own body, unable to move, touch, locomote, or groom. Proud men or women in a culture that makes a fetish of self-determination and independence may not be able to bear the thought of being incontinent of bowel and bladder or simply unable to answer the phone or use a toothbrush.

The answer from medicine to concerns about suffering so far has been silence. Even hospice has concentrated mainly on the management of pain, not suffering. But for many Americans it is suffering that is to be feared, that makes them concerned about quality of life, that gets them wondering about whether the cost is worth living, and it is suffering that leads many to think about ending their lives (Callahan, 1995). When one looks at the question of who wants the right to assistance in dying and why they want it, the answer is suffering. The concern to avoid suffering, broadly construed to include loss of dignity, self-esteem, and fear of dependency, is the strongest challenge hospice has ever faced (Shavelson, 1995).

For Many, Impairment Is Enough

Most people who favor changing the law to permit assistance in dying want to place tight restrictions on who will be granted this right. In the version of the law enacted in the State of Oregon, in the decisions of federal appellate courts, and in many articles and books, it is only the competent who are permitted to voluntarily elect to die with help from a doctor. One of the few who has shown no interest in restricting access to assistance in dying to the competent terminally ill is Dr. Jack Kevorkian. It is important to note how widespread support has been for his actions among both the public and in some quarters within the health professions despite his indifference to the issue of whether those requesting assisted suicide are actually terminally ill (Caplan, 1995a).

Kevorkian has always maintained that anyone who is competent should have the right to suicide assistance on demand. He has been willing to back this belief with action. At least three of the persons he assisted in dying were not terminally ill.

Limiting the right to assistance in dying to those who request it makes sense. After all, no one should be helped to die against his or her will. To kill without a request is murder, not suicide. Involuntary euthanasia, at the direction of family, doctors, or the state, is an especially morally suspect activity. The worst genocide in this century took place with the moral rationale that involuntary euthanasia of Jews, Gypsies, Jehovah's Witnesses, Communists, Slavs, persons with handicaps, and homosexuals was ethically justified (Caplan, 1992c).

But it is unlikely that assistance in dying is something that will long be restricted to the terminally ill. For too many Americans the issue of when to die involves neither terminal illness nor pain. It involves the loss of a sense of personal identity, the loss of dignity, and the loss of an acceptable quality of life. This is the group that poses the greatest challenge to the tradition of hospice, since many of those who fit these categories are not now and have not been candidates for eligibility for hospice. Yet they are strong candidates for requesting help in dying (Callahan, 1995).

Who Needs Assisted Suicide?

Most Americans are competent when they die. They can direct their doctors to use no aggressive means to prolong their dying. They can request and should receive all the pain control they wish. They should be permitted to leave the hospital and nursing home and return to their own home to die with assistance if they so choose. And they should not be forced to transfer from a nursing home or chronic care facility to die if they do not wish aggressive care at the end of life.

Living wills, DNR orders, advance directives, durable powers of attorney—all of these are the weapons that the competent have to control their dying. They can say no to any and all medical care. They may die where they wish. They may die pain free. Few among the ranks of the competent and dying will need any assistance from anybody in hastening their death.

Who then are the actual subjects of discussion if not the competent who are dying who need or might seek help in dying? It is those afflicted with terrible suffering, with challenges to their sense of independence and control, those who are fearful of losing their sense of self, and those who are too incompetent to do anything about the course of their care. In short, it is likely to be those who do view their lives as not worth living or who, if they could regain enough competency to see what has become of themselves, would most assuredly reject their fate if it involved living with their mental capacities, bodily functions, or both severely diminished or absent.

Those with advanced ALS, Parkinsonism, severe arthritis, Alzheimer's, chronic severe depression, severe burns, disfiguring injuries, brain injury, advanced cystic fibrosis, massive stroke, and many other disorders, diseases, and impairments will press for relief from their suffering. While the hospice movement has confined its attention to those facing imminent and certain death, these groups are not concerned with such limits. And their involvement in assisted suicide threatens to overwhelm both interest in and support for hospice as a prelude to dying under any circumstances.

It is also unlikely that restrictions requiring voluntary consent will withstand public pressure to permit some who are incompetent, such as terminally ill or severely disabled newborns and children, persons who are retarded or obviously mentally ill or impaired but who are severely restricted in their bodily functions and capacities, to obtain assistance in dying. Arguments for equal protection will quickly emerge as society increases its acceptance of assisted suicide as a response to suffering, broadly defined, within the competent population.

Consequences for Hospice

If autonomy is placed at the center of ethical discourse in a society, as it surely is in the United States, then it is very difficult to mount a persuasive argument against the legalization of assisted suicide by health care professionals. If it is true that self-determination includes the right to decide when life has become unbearable or burdensome and if it is also true that the only way to permit the safe and humane ending of life is through the participation of health care professionals, then the case for assisted suicide is not difficult to make on moral and political grounds.

It is a recognized fact that pain control is sometimes not what it ought to be for those who are dying and that even when pain can be controlled it sometimes requires rendering a person stuperous and incoherent, a state many find unacceptable. While those in the hospice movement may know that most cases of pain can be adequately controlled without severely impairing the cognitive capacities of the patient, it is nonetheless true that some persons will not wish to undergo a regimen of palliation while others would find their pain so severe that palliation will require putting them into states of mental functioning that are deemed unacceptable.

If a person believes that his or her quality of life has become so diminished, not as a result of pain but as a result of the suffering associated with disability, that it is unacceptably burdensome to live, the right to self-determination and control over one's fate seems also to point toward the right to assistance in dying. The loss of dignity associated with severely diminished function is often more than some people wish to bear. Hospice has little to offer to such persons.

Since no one is proposing involuntary euthanasia, nor is anyone calling for the mandatory invocation of assisted suicide for those who reach a given level of impairment, proponents of changing public policy need only note that they favor the creation of the option of assisted suicide. Legalization of assisted suicide may be a good even for those who choose not to take this path. The mere fact that the opportunity for help in dying exists may help some persons to endure more disability or dysfunction than they otherwise might have been willing to face (Shavelson, 1995).

Hospice has relatively little to say in the face of such arguments. Hospice workers can say that they are morally uncomfortable with assisting in dying, but such reservations do not directly meet the claim that respect for autonomy and humaneness requires making assisted suicide available performed by those willing to do so. Hospice advocates may say that hospice treatments and techniques can give hope to many facing imminent death, but that does not address the needs of those who find what goes on in a hospice unacceptable from their own view of dignity and self-control. And those with experience in hospice can say that they have seen many patients adapt and accommodate to the realities of infirmity and incapacity which may accompany dying, but again this is not an argument that will persuade those who maintain they ought be free to forgo these adaptive experiences if they so wish. And unless those in hospice are prepared to radically alter the prevailing criteria for admission, there will be some patients for whom hospice cannot be an option because they are not terminally ill but who see death as desirable owing to the burden of disease or impairment.

Hospice does not fare well placed against these positions. It does not meet the needs of many, and for some its very mode of treatment is unacceptable. While most people, even those who are very sick, may want to prolong their lives as much as they can, once a decision has been made to die, if the option exists to end life quickly, many will opt for this course rather then one of palliation, support, and pain control. If and when active euthanasia becomes public policy, existing hospice programs will either have to incorporate assisted dying into their care plans or risk elimination by new forms of terminal illness care which include assistance in dying for those who request it.

The only way hospice in the United States can avoid this scenario is to try to convince Americans that a good death is not one in which a life ends abruptly, at the first sign of pain or disability. Hospice, to remain as it is, must be able not just to provide support and palliative care but to convince people that these are the things they need as a part of the best possible death.

Those in hospice must also be able to persuade Americans that a good death can be a relatively cheap and affordable one. Many Americans fear the economic consequences of a high technology death. They do not want to spend their resources on treatments that are perceived to be of little benefit. Similarly, if hospice care is seen as expensive or burdensome to the patient or the patient's family, then the option of a planned death will loom as more attractive from the point of view of the bottom line, the patient's as well as society's. Again, the only hope hospice has of preserving its mission of providing support but not suicide to the terminally ill is to be able to make a persuasive case that a hospice-mediated death is a good death and one that is worth the cost to the patient, the patient's family, and society.

I am not sure that even these steps will be sufficient to preserve the mission and philosophy of hospice as they now exist. The creation of a right to die on demand with the aid of a doctor or a nurse may simply make hospice appear to be an anachronism in the eyes of many who might once have considered it as a way to die. Hospice arose as a way to ensure a good death in a medical system overly obsessed with utilizing expensive high technology upon the dying. If it is to endure, hospice must be able to explain why the kind of death it provides is an attractive and affordable alternative to a quick, cheap, and easy death at the hands of a health care professional.

eight

Odds and Ends

MUCH OF WHAT PASSES FOR METHODOLOGY in bioethics goes under the name of conceptual analysis. To put the point another way, bioethicists spend a lot of their time arguing about the precise meanings of words. Those having neither the temperament nor the patience for undertaking or pondering the results of this type of verbal dissection use rather less flattering albeit more colorful descriptions of the activity, descriptions in which images of heads located in clouds, dances conducted around the heads of pins, or the products of bovine excretion loom large. The ongoing wrangling about the concept of medical futility (Misbin et al., 1995) is a perfect example of why some find bioethics valuable whereas others do not.

On the plus side, careful analysis of the concept of medical futility has produced a number of crucial insights with immediate practical application. Medical futility must be understood as referring both to the probability of attaining a particular diagnostic, therapeutic, or palliative goal and to the desirability of attaining that goal (Schneiderman et al., 1990, 1995, 1996). Practitioners must be alert to both dimensions in dealing with patients, colleagues, students, and families.

On the minus side, analysis of the concept has produced no consensus about how it should be defined or used. Various analysts who have gone to the plate and taken mighty swings at defining futility find themselves disagreeing about how sound probability estimates of the success to be expected from particular treatments are or can ever be (Rubenfeld and Crawford, 1996; Faber-Langendoen et al., 1993; Christakis and Asch, 1993), who should be involved in making estimates about the chances for success (Schneiderman et al., 1996; Halevy and Brody, 1996), what value ought be assigned to the attainment of particular goals for particular patients (Misbin et al., 1995; Schneiderman et al., 1996; Halevy and Brody, 1996; Truog et al., 1992), and how to implement policies which invoke medical futility (Misbin et al., 1995; Halevy and Brody, 1996).

An assessment of the struggle to define and operationalize a concept as freighted with moral baggage as medical futility runs the risk of seeming, well, futile. The disputants are far apart in their thinking.

When keening their loudest, proponents of the utility of futility, aptly described as futilitarians (Schneiderman et al., 1990, 1995, 1996; Rubenfeld and Crawford, 1996; Faber-Langendoen et al., 1993), see nothing less than the demise of the profession of medicine if doctors refuse to do what is futile. Professional integrity requires that physicians say, on the basis of evidence, expertise, and clinical experience, that some medical interventions for some patients are pointless, useless, and meaningless.

The critics bay back that integrating medical futility into clinical practice is at best immoral, in that doctors have no grounds for imposing on patients their personal values about what odds or ends are worth pursuing (Misbin et al., 1995; Schneiderman et al., 1996; Truog et al., 1992), and at worse misleading, since statistical information about classes of patients frequently cannot be used to forecast the outcome faced by any particular patient.

It is hard not to take sides in such a spirited debate, especially when the pages of prominent journals are open to publishing yet one more round. It is hard, but it is the right thing to do.

One lesson quickly learned by anyone who engages in conceptual analysis of a bioethical problem is that a concept should not be asked to bear more weight than it can reasonably sustain. I am afraid that is what has happened to medical futility.

Proponents of the utility of medical futility (Schneiderman et al., 1996) are correct in arguing that information about the likelihood of producing various treatment outcomes can and must be of central importance in the practice of medicine. It is possible, as recent studies show (Rubenfeld and Crawford, 1996), to use retrospective case history analysis to identify predictors of death and mortality trends associated with treatments provided to various categories of patient. The longstanding lament by policymakers, third-party payers, and consumers and providers of health care that far too little in the practice of medicine rests upon evidence-based outcome standards (Office of Technology Assessment, 1994) imposes a duty to collect and utilize information about treatment outcomes, including especially death, the inability to exist without technological life support being given in an intensive care unit, and the inability to restore consciousness. These end points are all key elements in any plausible definition of medical futility (Schneiderman et al., 1990, 1995, 1996; Faber-Langendoen et al., 1993).

The problem confronting futilitarians is not one of definition. While there are always gray zones, the medical profession is free to be somewhat stipulative and arbitrary about odds and ends in publicly setting out boundaries for futility. Courts, legislatures, patient advocacy groups, and the media quickly challenge any limit that appears overly arbitrary or restrictive. Any doubts about our society's wariness of talk of limits should evaporate in the face of the mini-maelstroms that have surrounded efforts to test the efficacy of salvage chemotherapy and bone marrow transplant for end-stage breast cancer and heart and lung reduction surgery for these failing organs. Even in the absence of any evidence that these treatments work, there has been enormous pressure to include them among the things insurance companies, government programs, and managed care organizations must cover.

The problem facing those who put their hope in medical futility as a way to rationalize the provision of care is not the lack of consensus about a definition. Instead it is the absence of trust between doctor and patient when it comes to weighing odds and ends.

Without trust, outcomes-based medicine is doomed. If patient and family are going to trust the pronouncement of a physician that there is no point in continuing mechanical ventilation past a fixed number of days after a bone marrow transplant (Rubenfeld and Crawford, 1996; Faber-Langendoen, 1991) or that there is no hope of recovery no matter what is done for a child born with anencephaly (Caplan, 1995a), they must first trust the doctor. Numbers alone, even staggeringly grim ones derived from thousands of cases and years of experience, will not suffice. Dry figures turn to dust in the face of desperation. Trust is the only tool the doctor has to persuade a patient that a long shot, an innovative idea, or something touted in a grocery store supermarket tabloid is not worth trying. However, trust between doctor and patient and doctor and family is in jeopardy in medicine today.

A major source of distrust between doctors and patients is medicine's continued inability to break down the barriers posed by race, ethnicity, religion, and economic disparity (Witzig, 1996; Connors and Smith,

1996). When patients do not trust what the doctor says, not for want of evidence about prognosis and benefit but because they do not believe the physician is their advocate because the doctor does things that are racially or culturally insensitive, shows little or no interest in their religious beliefs (Connors and Smith, 1996), or simply seems too distant and removed from their own lived experience, the prognosis for following the doctor's advice is poor. When patients have no health insurance or cannot meet the requirements for co-payment, they have reason to wonder when the doctor says all that can be done has been done. When the doctor says he or she has no idea whom the patient should talk with to obtain spiritual support or emotional sustenance, then trust cannot flourish. When the prognosis for trust is poor, the prospects for guiding treatment by means of data concerning medical futility are, to put a number on them, zero.

Part of the reason that numbers cannot shape clinical care is that patients and families are not interested in numbers; they are interested in hope. Moreover, they are interested in doing those things that show they are brave, courageous fighters, loyal and steadfast. To forgo any chance at cure may appear to compromise these interests. What parents would sleep well at night knowing they had willingly forgone a one-in-a-million chance to save their baby? How many daughters could say to their mothers that the odds of survival are so remote that they think it best to stop care? Who among us, wanting to make sure that our family and friends think well of us, can say as we die that we are giving in to illness and disease and will not put up a fight? Quitting is hardly a virtue in American society.

Add to this mix the current efforts to contain costs that put the physician under a duty to consider not only patient needs but also the fiscal consequences of the provision of care. Could any mix be more corrosive of trust?

If physicians are not seen as zealous advocates for the interests of those in their care, then a certain degree of skepticism will attend any pronouncement of medical futility (Caplan, 1997a, 1997b). Organizational and payment schemes that threaten advocacy at the bedside undermine the willingness of patients and families to trust in the statements about odds and ends that doctors make (Mechanic and Schlesinger, 1996).

Futilitarians are right to urge that medicine pay more attention to outcomes and use this information to guide the care provided to patients. However, they are wrong to place all their hopes on finding an explication of medical futility that will win the day. The prognosis for medical futility's becoming a more central part of the practice of medicine hinges on what medicine does to cement trust with those in its care. When the doctor is seen as someone who has the moral authority to say enough is enough and who can provide the emotional support to go along with throwing in the towel or at least locate that support for those who need it, then and only then will data about futility assume a more central role in clinical practice. The greater the trust between doctor and patient, the more willing Americans will be to accept not pursuing long odds to achieve bad ends.

PART THREE

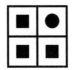

TRANSPLANTATION

nine

No Sale:
Markets, Organs,
and Tissues

THE UNITED STATES IS AWASH IN A SEA of proposals calling for the creation of financial incentives as the solution to the shortage of cadaver organs and tissues available to those requiring transplants (Buttle, 1991; Carson, 1996; Cohen, 1989, 1992; Hansmann, 1989; Harvey, 1990; Peters, 1991a, b; National Kidney Foundation, 1991; UNOS Update, 1991; Wright, 1995; Williams, 1995). Even Dr. Jack Kevorkian has weighed in on the side of auctioning off body parts as the way to solve the gap between supply and demand in transplantation (Kevorkian, 1992). Although these proposals vary in the details of how payment might be implemented, the supposition they have in common is that monetary incentives will increase organ donation.

While those bellowing for markets in parts think that the road to abundance in vital organs runs through your wallet, there is a special interest in using money to lure the poor into the world of organ supply. The primary targets of financial compensation in many of the plans, sometimes explicitly acknowledged as such (Peters, 1991b, UNOS Update, 1991), are African Americans. Studies show that blacks do not donate organs at the same rate as whites and have not for some time

(Callender, 1987). Proponents of fiscal rewards argue that since minorities are more likely to be poor, financial incentives are likely to be disproportionately attractive to them.

Since poor people confronting death sometimes also face the prospect of uncovered medical expenses, funeral costs, or both for themselves or their deceased loved ones, proponents of paying for organs argue that they and their families can be swayed by money to make organs and tissues available. The advocates for financial incentives claim that these costs are a burden for indigent families and that empathy for their impoverished plight justifies the creation of compensation schemes.

The fact that money is omnipresent in transplantation really gets the juices flowing among advocates of open markets in body parts. Proponents sometimes suggest that paying money for body parts makes sense, since other parties, from procurement organizations to transplant surgeons, make money from transplantation. Why should patients and families be the only ones left out of the financial bonanza that transplantation represents? It is simply unfair and even a bit of a scam. It should be legal for potential sources and their families, especially poor persons and their families, to be compensated and share in the bounty that is transplantation.

I believe that any form of compensation for cadaver organs and tissues is immoral. A national policy, regional efforts, or pilot projects permitting compensation for cadaver organs and tissues, either in a direct or indirect manner, would have deleterious consequences for those currently awaiting organ and tissue transplants in the United States. The factual grounds for thinking that money will lead to a significant increase in cadaver organ and tissue availability, either among the general population or the poor, do not exist. Moreover, there are serious ethical reasons for not permitting financial rewards to be associated with cadavers.

No factual support has been advanced for the hypothesis that payment will increase cadaver donation. What passes for evidence about what motivates people to be donors can most generously be described as vapid bias. There is no empirical evidence that families raise the issue of money or compensation at the time when they are faced with requests or decisions about making organs and tissues available for transplantation. What factual evidence is available lends support to the opposite conclusion—that significant numbers of Americans would be angered, offended, and insulted by offers of money or financial rewards for the organs and tissues of their deceased loved ones (Caplan and Virnig, 1990; Davis, 1991; Watts, 1991; Siminoff et al., 1995).

A variety of state, federal, professional, and international organizations and societies have repeatedly prohibited and condemned any form of commerce in cadaver organs. The consistent rejection by legislative groups, courts, and professional organizations of compensation schemes illustrates the depth of public opposition to paying for cadaveric remains (Task Force on Organ Transplantation, 1986; *Moore v. Regents,* 1990; National Organ Transplant Act, 1984; World Health Organization, 1991).

Almost forty years of public policy must be considered in weighing the likely impact of any deviation from the existing system of voluntary donation as the basis of cadaver organ and tissue procurement (Caplan, Siminoff, Arnold, and Virnig, 1992; Siminoff et al., 1995). During the past three decades, massive educational and public service campaigns have been undertaken to urge organ and tissue donation. Health care professionals and the public have repeatedly been told that the "gift of life" is to be made solely on the basis of altruistic, voluntary choice (Youngner et al., 1989). Since the language of donation and gift giving is completely incompatible with any system that provides fiscal rewards only for those who actually make organs and tissues available when death occurs, any scheme calling for compensation will offend those who have come to believe that money and cadaver procurement do not and should not mix.

The argument that financial incentives would be especially attractive to the poor and would thus help redress the underrepresentation of African Americans and other minorities in the existing donor pool sounds persuasive in the abstract. But only in the abstract. A public policy of money for body parts is inexcusably indifferent to the history of African Americans and slavery in this and other countries. It is likely that African Americans would find such a policy morally offensive for reasons of history. Having fought for decades to escape the legacy of slavery, there might well be limited enthusiasm for proposals that permit sales of body organs to wealthy people willing to pony up for parts postmortem.

If the only way U.S. society, or any other, can find to pay for the uncompensated costs of medical care or funerals for the indigent is to offer cash for their body parts, such a society has no right to call itself humane, decent, or fair. Unless those on waiting lists are allowed to pay whatever the market will bear, the burdens of poverty will continue to be present for the indigent. But the poor will not be allowed to sell cadaveric organs and tissues to the highest bidder, since this would undoubtedly result in prices that would make the costs of transplantation even more prohibitive then they already are. The poor are not likely to see their poverty much alleviated by permitting limited or unlimited organ and tissue sale. In nations where markets have been allowed or tolerated—India, the Philippines, and Brazil, for example—the market in body parts has done little to advance the interests of the poor.

What is worse, arguing for markets and sales in the name of the poor puts medicine in an untenable moral position. It seems to be favoring a shift in public policy which suggests that medicine's only obligation to alleviate the plight of the poor is to those willing to sign over their organs and tissues for transplantation. Or, to put it bluntly, unless you are selling your liver or bone marrow, your funeral is your funeral. Since the current crop of plans call for compensation to be provided only for families that consent to sell, mewing about empathy for the plight of the poor as the motive to legitimate markets has the distinctively hollow ring of hypocrisy.

Paying for organs and tissues is especially offensive at a time when so many poor people face fiscal obstacles to receiving transplants. Access to transplants is all too real a problem for the poor and for minorities (Caplan, 1989c, 1992; Ubel and Caplan, 1997; United States General Accounting Office, 1989). The transplant community in particular and the medical community in general should not accept a scheme which permits payment for organs and tissues when financial hurdles make access to transplants impossible for too many of the poor. Would the poor and minority communities accept for long the cruel irony of being less likely to be able to afford but more likely to be available to sell body parts? Before calling for markets or compensation for cadaver parts, the transplant community and organized medicine at least have an obligation to ensure that every American in need has an equal chance to receive a transplant.

Financial incentives reduce people to merchandise. Offering bribes, permitting cash rebates, setting estate discounts, or paying for funerals contingent on a favorable decision about procurement says that medicine is willing to commodify the body to whatever extent it takes to allow more transplants to be done. Organ donors cannot be paid and still be donors. Those whose organs and tissues are taken in the context of financial reward become sources not donors (Marshall, Thomasma, and Daar, 1996).

Payment for the bodies of the dead carries special moral significance for African Americans in light of U.S. history. African Americans for hundreds of years suffered the horror of being bought and sold as chattel. As slaves, their bodies were often used by physicians without consent for experimentation and after death for autopsy and teaching purposes (Savitt, 1982). Their attitudes about payment for organs and tissues are likely to be influenced by the historical reality of slavery in a way that none of those calling for markets and compensation have acknowledged, much less taken into account. It is of no small significance to many African Americans that the last time the federal government paid for funeral expenses for poor African Americans was when their bodies were sought for autopsy in the notorious Tuskegee syphilis study (Brandt, 1978; Jones, 1981; also see chapter 2). Payment for the body is more likely to offend and outrage the sensibilities of the African American community than it is to encourage participation as sources of organs and tissues after death.

Calls for payment for body parts also ignore the fragile nature of support among religious organizations for cadaveric procurement. Historically, some major religious faiths have had reservations and doubts about the moral licitness of transplantation (Wolstenholme and O'Conner, 1968; May, 1988; John Paul II, 1991). They have supported the use of cadaver organs only insofar as the practice is seen as humane, respectful of the deceased, and treating the body neither as property nor a commodity. Proposals permitting sale or reimbursement only when organs and tissues are made available from the dead inevitably require the body to be viewed as subject to ownership and commerce. As such, they are very likely to encounter sustained and vigorous opposition from many religious leaders (John Paul II, 1991).

Some say we should at least give financial incentives a chance by trying pilot programs in some areas of the country (Peters, 1991a; National Kidney Foundation, 1991). Such proposals are naive. It is absurd to believe that the practice of paying for organs in one part of the country will not affect the donation process in other areas. In fact, in countries such as India, Brazil and the Philippines, the practice of paying living unrelated donors has had a negative influence on cadaver donation (Kandela, 1991), and there is no reason to believe that it would be otherwise here.

The practical problems of implementing financial incentives for cadaver organs and tissues are enormous. If reimbursement were legal, it would not be long before the prices sought and paid either aboveboard or on the black market escalated. If, on the other hand, buyers were allowed to set their price, then financial incentive schemes would disenfranchise and disadvantage the interests of the very groups often cited by those advancing fiscal schemes, indigent recipients awaiting transplants, since they would not be able to compete for cadaveric parts in a market.

If compensation is allowed, will donors or physicians be financially liable if they decide that certain donors are medically unsuitable as sources, thereby preventing a poor person from making money? Would they be liable for failing at efforts to detect and pronounce brain death or for waiting too long to declare death, thereby costing relatives their chance at a pot of gold from the distribution of the deceased's remains? Who will pay for brain-death protocols to be carried out when families insist some effort be made to see whether procurement might be possible? How long will it be before funeral directors, medical examiners, coroners, and procurement personnel begin to seek payment according to what the market will bear for their roles in cadaver organ and tissue procurement?

Practical and technical problems, however, are not the main reason for opposing financial reimbursement for making organs and tissues available after death. Calls for markets, compensation, bounties, or rewards should be rejected because they convert human beings into products, a metaphysical transformation that cheapens the respect for life and corrodes our ability to maintain the stance that human beings are special, unique, and valuable for their own sake, not for what others can mine, extract, or manufacture from them. Nor will markets do what their proponents hope. The inevitable opposition such proposals will encounter from many religious leaders means any increase in lives saved attributable to cash prizes will be swamped by the number of lives lost when those who refuse to see the human body as available for sale decline to participate in anything having to do with transplants. When aimed primarily at increasing the supply of organs and tissues from African Americans, proposals to market are so indifferent to the symbolism that treating the body as an object of commerce has for the members of that community that their failure is certain.

Once the decision is made to pay for human parts, all that is left is haggling about the price. The human body should not be made the subject of haggling. Proposals to permit fiscal incentives in organ and tissue procurement should be rejected. The consequences of commercializing ourselves in terms of lives lost and values compromised is too high a price to pay.

ten

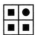

Is the Use of Animal Organs for Transplants Immoral?

IT IS TEMPTING TO THINK THAT A DECISION about whether or not it is immoral to use animals as sources for transplantable organs and tissues hinges only upon the question of whether or not it is safe to use their parts. In the past few years the debate about whether a baboon or a chimp should be slaughtered in order to obtain its liver or bone marrow has hinged almost exclusively on the question of whether or not terrible diseases might inadvertently be transferred from animals to people. So terrifying is the prospect of somehow transferring a strange new disease to the recipient of an animal organ and then on to the rest of humanity that nearly every commission that has been asked to examine the ethics of xenografting has focused on only this issue (FDA, 1996; Nuffield, 1996; IOM, 1996).

The ethics of xenografting, however, involves more than an analysis of that question. The assessment should begin with the morality of killing animals to obtain their parts. And even this basic question, which of necessity precedes the safety issue, is more complicated than it might at first glance appear to be.

In order to decide whether it is ethical to kill animals, a variety of subsidiary questions must be considered. Is it ethical to kill animals in order to obtain organs and tissues to save human lives or alleviate severe disability when it might not be ethical to kill them for food or sport

(Singer, 1975, 1992, 1995)? Why are animals being considered as sources of organs and tissues—do alternative methods for obtaining replacement parts for human beings exist? What sorts of animals would have to be killed, how would they be killed, and how would they be stored, handled, and treated prior to their deaths?

If it is possible to defend the killing of animals for xenografting, then questions as to the morality of subjecting human beings to the risks, both physical and psychological, associated with xenografting must also be weighed. In undertaking a xenograft on a human subject, the focus of moral concern ought not be solely on the animal that will be sacrificed.

Even for persons who eat meat or hunt, it might well seem immoral to kill animals for their parts if alternative sources of replacement parts were or might soon be available. The moral acceptability of xenografting will for many, including the prospective recipients of animal parts, be contingent on the presumption that there is no other plausible alternative source of transplantable organs and tissues. Unfortunately, the scarcity that is behind the current interest in xenografting is all too real.

Why Pursue Xenografting?

The supply of organs and tissues available from human cadaver sources for transplantation in the United States and other nations is entirely inadequate. Many children and adults die or remain disabled owing to the shortage of transplantable organs and tissues. Unless a solution is found to the problem of scarcity, the plight of those in need of organs and tissues will only grow worse, and the numbers who die solely for want of an organ will continue to grow.

More than a third of those now awaiting liver transplants die for want of a donor organ. Well over half of all children born with fatal congenital deformities of the heart or liver die without a transplant because of the shortage of available organs. The percentage of those who die while waiting would actually be higher if all potential candidates were on waiting lists (Baum et al., 1991).

Some Americans are not referred for transplants because they cannot afford them. If those from economically underdeveloped nations with organ failure were wait-listed at North American and European transplant centers, the percentage of those who die while awaiting a transplant would be much larger (Caplan, 1989c).

More than 150,000 Americans with kidney failure are kept alive by renal dialysis. The cost for this treatment exceeded $5 billion in 1997. It would be far cheaper and, from the patient's quality-of-life perspective, far more desirable to treat kidney failure by means of transplants. There are, however, simply not enough cadaver kidneys for all who desire and could benefit from a transplant.

The supply of cadaver organs for pancreas, small intestine, lung, or heart-lung transplants is not adequate to the demand posed by those dying from a wide variety of diseases affecting these organs. The same story holds for bone, ligament, dural matter, heart valves, and skin. Moreover, demand for the limited supply of organs and tissues is increasing as more and more medical centers become capable of offering this form of surgery and as techniques for managing rejection and infection improve (Caplan et al., 1992).

The shortage of organs and tissues for transplantation has led researchers to pursue a variety of alternatives in order to bridge the gap between supply and demand. Some suggest changing existing public policies governing cadaver procurement. Others focus on locating alternatives to human cadaver organs.

Efforts could be made to modify public policy to encourage more persons to serve as organ and tissue donors. Legislation mandating that the option of organ and tissue donation be presented whenever a person dies in a hospital setting has been enacted in the United States, but while it has led to increases in both tissue and organ availability, those asking find themselves confronting a high number of refusals (Caplan and Virnig, 1990; Caplan, 1991; Siminoff et al., 1995). A significant degree of mistrust and misunderstanding about donation on the part of the public still exists (Caplan, 1991).

Other proposals involve changing laws to permit payment to those who agree to donate or whose families consent to cadaver donation (see chapter 9 and Peters, 1991a; Wight, 1991) and moving toward a presumed consent system in which those who do not wish to donate would have to carry cards or other evidence of their nondonor status. However, cultural and religious attitudes in large segments of the U.S. and other societies will not support the creation of markets, bounties, or property status for body parts (John Paul II, 1991) or the extension of state authority to the seizure of cadaver organs and tissues.

Allowing markets may lead to criminal activities (*New Scientist,* 1991). Selling irreplaceable body parts is an especially repugnant way to ask a person to earn income or benefits (Tufts, 1991). There is much reluctance on the part of the general public to swap the presumption of individual control over the body, either in life or death, for a policy that might benefit the common good by risking the loss of personal autonomy (Tufts, 1991; Caplan et al., 1992). Nor has the actual experience with presumed consent laws in European nations been such as to justify enthusiasm for the likely results of a shift away from individualism and personal autonomy with respect to the control of cadavers (Eurotransplant Foundation, 1991).

Even if drastic changes were made in existing public policies, other factors are working against the prospects for large increases in the human cadaver organ supply. Improvements in emergency room access and care, the AIDS epidemic, ambivalence about cadaver donation on the part of the public, plus laudable advances in public health measures such as mandatory seatbelt use, raising the age for legally purchasing liquor, and tougher laws against drunk driving mean that a tremendous increase in the supply of cadaver organs is unlikely to occur no matter what public policies are adopted.

Most important with respect to the moral defensibility of exploring xenografting as an alternative source of organs, the supply would still not meet the potential demand even if all human cadaver organs were somehow made available for transplant. The hidden pool of potential transplant recipients would quickly become visible were these organs and tissues to become available (Caplan, 1989c, 1991). The search for alternatives to the use of human cadaver organs rests on the recognition that scarcity is an insurmountable obstacle.

In recent years, surgeons have tried to solve the problem of shortage by using kidneys as well as segments of liver, lung and pancreas from living donors. Transplant teams in a few nations have been testing the feasibility of transplanting lobes of livers between biologically related individuals (Raia, Nery, and Mies, 1989; Strong et al., 1990). Teams at Stanford University and the University of Minnesota, among others, have used parents as lung donors for their children. Minnesota and other centers have been experimenting for many years with transplants of the kidney and segments of the pancreas from related and unrelated living donors (Elick et al., 1990). Many centers around the world have performed bone marrow transplants between biologically unrelated persons.

There are serious problems with and limits to the use of living donors as alternative sources of organs and tissues (see chapter 11). No transplant center would use a living person as a heart donor for another on the grounds that it is immoral to kill one person to save another. Using living donors for other organs requires subjecting the donors to life-threatening risks, some pain and disfigurement, and some risk of disability. The legitimacy of consent on the part of living donors, especially among family members, is hard to assess. And since it is not known whether transplanting lobes or segments of organs or unrelated bone marrow is efficacious, it is not certain that this strategy for getting more organs and tissue is a realistic option, much less whether it will prove attractive to a sufficient number of actual donors.

Another alternative to human cadaver organ transplantation is the development of mechanical or artificial organ and tissue substitutes. Kidney dialysis is one such substitute. The widely publicized efforts to create a total artificial heart, first at the University of Utah and then at Humana Audubon Hospital in Louisville, Kentucky (see chapter 3), represent another albeit failed effort to create an alternative to transplantation using cadaver hearts. New generations of mechanical hearts are in the research pipeline, as are artificial insulin pumps, artificial lungs, and various types of artificial livers. Safe, effective, and reliable artificial organs and tissues, however, still appear to be decades away.

Ironically, even those artificial organs that are currently available increase rather than decrease the problem of allocating the small number of organs available for transplants. These devices permit transplant teams to temporarily "bridge" children and adults who would otherwise die by putting them on devices such as left ventricular assist devices, heart-lung machines, extracorporeal membrane oxygenators, liquid ventilation, and artificial livers which are either too unsafe or too damaging to the health of the recipient to allow long-term or permanent use. Bridging those with organ failure using mechanical devices increases the pool of prospective recipients. There are more potential recipients than there otherwise might have been had bridging not been possible. In fact, not only are there larger numbers of persons competing for the same relatively small supply of organs, but under criteria which favor medical urgency, bridge recipients often receive the highest priority in gaining access to transplants. This is so even though evidence, particularly with respect to liver and kidney transplants, shows that persons on mechanical support do not do as well in terms of survival after a transplant as those who were not so critically ill.

It is the plight of those dying from end-stage diseases for want of donor organs from both living and cadaver human sources that has led a number of research groups to explore the option of using animals as the source of transplantable organs and tissues. Transplant researchers at Loma Linda, Duke, Pittsburgh, Stanford, Columbia, and Minnesota as well as in England, China, Belgium, Sweden, Japan, and France, among other countries, are conducting research on xenografting organs and tissues. Some are exploring the feasibility of primate-to-human transplants. Others are pursuing lines of research that would allow them to use animals other than primates as sources. And some are especially interested in using specially bred genetically engineered animals such as pigs to supply organs to humans.

It is scarcity that grounds the moral case for thinking about animals as sources of organs and tissues. In light of current and potential demand, no other options exist for alleviating the scarcity in the supply of replacement parts. If, however, society were to decide not to perform transplants or to perform only a limited number of them, then the case for xenografting would be considerably weakened. While transplant surgeons and those on waiting lists may find strategies for finding more organs or tissues attractive, another possible response to scarcity is to simply live with it. Those who advocate this response could do so on the grounds that it is not morally necessary to perform transplants on all persons who are in need, especially if doing so requires the systematic sacrifice of animals for human purposes (Regan and Singer, 1976; Singer, 1975; Caplan, 1985, 1992a).

What about Other Strategies?

It is possible to argue that the answer to the problem of scarcity in lieu of pursuing the option of xenografting is that medicine should simply stop doing transplants entirely or only do as many as can be done with whatever human cadaver organs and tissues are available. This moral stance might rest on the claim that transplants are simply too expensive and do not work well enough to justify a hunt for alternative sources to human organs. Or someone might view xenografting as unnecessary and immoral on the grounds that prevention makes far more sense than salvage and rescue in dealing with end-stage organ failure. Some forms of transplantation are notoriously expensive. A critic of the xenografting option might argue that it is not wise to spend hundreds of thousands of dollars on heart, liver, or nonrelated bone marrow transplants when the number of people requiring these treatments could be drastically reduced by decreasing the incidence of smoking, alcohol consumption, and exposure to toxic substances in the workplace and the environment.

The arguments in favor of the "live within your means" position are not persuasive. While prevention of organ and tissue failure is surely to be preferred to rescue by means of transplants, large numbers of persons suffer organ and tissue failure for reasons that are poorly understood and thus not amenable to prevention. While individuals should certainly be encouraged to adopt more healthful lifestyles (including the consumption of less animal fat), there are no proven techniques available for ensuring that people will behave wisely or prudently. Moreover, those who will need transplants in the next few decades are persons for whom prevention is too late. So while prevention is desirable, the demand for transplants will not diminish for a significant period regardless of the efforts undertaken to improve public health.

Transplants are expensive, but many types of transplantation, especially for children and young adults, are very effective and provide a good quality of life for many years. The wisdom of doing any medical procedure cannot simply be equated with its overall cost. A more reasonable measure would be to see what is purchased for the price that is charged. If the moral value of spending money for health services is not total price but cost per year of life saved or cost relative to the likelihood of saving a life, then there are many other areas of health care that ought to be restricted or abandoned long before accepted forms of transplantation such as heart, liver, and kidney are deemed too expensive or not cost-worthy.

Ethical Problems with the Xenograft Option

If it is true that the case for pursuing xenografting is persuasive, then the question of whether xenografting is morally wrong shifts to an analysis of the type of animals to be used, the manner of their maintenance, and the risks and dangers involved for potential human recipients. Xenografting is still evolving, so the ethical issues must be considered under two broad headings: issues associated with basic and clinical experimentation and, if this proves successful, issues associated with the widespread use of xenografts as therapies.

RESEARCH ISSUES

In thinking about the ethics of research on xenografting, a couple of assumptions can safely be made. The number and type of animals used will be very much a function of cost, prior knowledge of the species, inbred characteristics, ease in handling, and availability. Gorillas are not going to be used in research, simply because there are too few of them and they are unlikely to make compliant subjects. Rats and mice will dominate the early stages of research (as they already do) because they are relatively well understood, special-purpose bred, and cheap to acquire and maintain. Few primates will be used for basic or clinical research simply because they are too scarce, too expensive, and too complex to permit controlled study for most experimental purposes.

Even if the number of animals to be used is relatively small, the question still must be faced as to whether it is ethical to use animal models involving species such as rats, chickens, sheep, pigs, monkeys, baboons, and chimps in order to study the feasibility of cross-species xenografting.

In part, the answer to this question pivots on whether or not there are plausible alternative models to the use of animals for exploring the two critical steps required for successful xenografting—overcoming immunological rejection and achieving long-term physiological function in an organ or tissue. To some extent, immunological problems can be examined without sacrificing primates or higher animals by using lower animals or cellular models. But there would not appear to be any viable alternatives or nonhuman substitutes available for understanding the processes involved in rejection. At best it may be possible to use animals that have fewer cognitive and intellectual capacities for most forms of basic research with respect to understanding the immunology of xenografting.

When research gets closer to the clinical stage, especially when it becomes possible to examine the extent to which xenografted organs and tissues can function posttransplant, it will be necessary to use some animals as donors and recipients that are closely related to human beings. If, in light of the scarcity of human organs, it is ethical to pursue the option of xenografting, then it would be unethical to subject human beings to any form of xenografting that has not undergone a prior demonstration of both immunological and physiological feasibility in animals closely analogous to humans.

The use of animals analogous to humans for basic research on xenografting means that some form of primates must be used both as donors and as recipients. Is it ethical to sacrifice primates, even if only a small number, to demonstrate the feasibility of xenografting in human beings? If primates and people have the same moral status, then it is hard to see how the use of primates could be justified (Regan and Singer, 1976; Regan and VanDeVeer, 1982; Singer, 1975, 1995). But are humans and apes moral equivalents?

At this point, those who want to deny the validity of moral equivalence begin to look for morally significant properties uniquely present in human beings but not in primates. Strong candidates for the property that might make a moral difference sufficient to allow the killing of primates to advance human interests are language, tool use, rationality, intentionality, consciousness, conscience, and/or empathy. The debate about the morality of sacrificing a primate of some sort to advance human interests by saving human lives then hinges on empirical facts about what a particular species of primate can or cannot do in comparison to what humans are capable of doing (Jasper and Nelkin, 1992).

It is indisputable that there are differences in the capacities and abilities of humans and primates. Chimps can sign, but humans have much more to say. Gorillas seem to reason, but humans have calculus, novels, and quantum theory. Humans are capable of a much broader range of behavior and intellectual functioning than is any other primate species.

Many who would protest the use of primates in xenografting research are keen to illustrate that primates possess many of the properties and abilities that are found to contribute moral standing to humans. The fact, however, that one species or another of primate is capable of some degree of intellectual or behavioral ability that seems worthy of moral respect when manifest by humans does not mean that human beings are the moral equivalents of other primates. It is one thing to argue that primates ought to have moral standing. It is a very different matter to argue that humans and other primates are morally equivalent. One can grant that primates deserve moral consideration without conceding that, on average, the death of a human being is of greater moral significance than is the death of a baboon, a green monkey, or a chimpanzee.

Xenografting involving primates can be morally justified on the grounds that, in general, human beings possess capacities and abilities that confer more moral value upon them than do the capacities of other primates and other animals. To believe that human beings have special moral worth is not a form of "speciesism" (Singer, 1975, 1992) but rather a claim of comparative worth based upon important empirical differences between classes of creatures.

There are empirical reasons to support the claim that it is worth sacrificing primates for humans or, for that matter, other animals for humans. As a group, humans have properties that confer greater moral worth and standing upon them than do other animal species. But the difference does not involve the hunt for some magical attribute or property that characterizes humans but animals lack. Rather it is the attributes of humans in the group or social form that distinguish them from other primates and other creatures. Human beings can be ethical. They may act this way only rarely and some may never do so, but we are creatures capable of moral activity and moral responsibility. Humans can be moral agents, while animals, even other primates, are moral subjects.

Animals have moral worth. Their suffering and intelligence make it intrinsically wrong to kill them for fun, sport, or pleasure or for no reason at all. But animals are incapable of being held to account for what they do. Your dog may soil the rug and a gorilla may attack its keeper, but these are not culpable or even moral choices. Only creatures with the capacity for culture, language, sociality, and conscience can live in a moral world in which moral agency is possible. It is the social attributes of humanity that confer more worth on its members than the baboon troop, the lion pride, or a gaggle of geese has.

Even conceding a difference in moral worth between humans and other species, there is still a problem when it comes to the sacrifice of an animal to save a person. Those who remain uninspired by the loftier worth I allege for humanity might ask whether scientists and surgeons should be willing to kill a retarded child or an adult in a permanent vegetative state in the service of saving lives.

It is indisputable that human beings have on average more capacities and abilities than do animals. But some individual animals, many of them primates, have more capacities and abilities than certain individual human beings who lack them due to congenital disorders or as the result of disease or injury. If it is argued that we ought to use animals instead of humans to assess the feasibility of xenografting because humans are more highly developed in terms of intellectual and emotional capacities, capacities that make a moral difference in that they are the basis for moral agency, then why should we not use a severely retarded child instead of a bright chimp or gorilla (Singer, 1992, 1995) as subjects in basic or clinical research? Unless those who are doing or wish to engage in basic research on xenografting can answer this question, they will be open to the charge of immorality.

One line of response is to simply say that we are powerful and the primates are less so; therefore they must yield to human purposes if we choose to experiment upon them rather than upon retarded children. This line of response, however, is far removed from the kinds of arguments that should be mustered in the name of morality. A more promising line of argument requires examining the issue head on to see why it is that it would be wrong to use a severely retarded child or a comatose person instead of a chimp in basic research or as a source of vital organs.

Two reasons might be given for picking a chimp instead of a human being with very limited or irreversibly damaged capacities. We might decide not to use a human being who has lost capacities and abilities out of respect for his or her former existence. If a person makes a conscious, deliberate, and voluntary decision to allow his or her body to be used for scientific research prior to becoming comatose, severely disabled, or brain dead, then those wishes could be honored and a moral case made that they should be. But if no such advance notice has been given, then we ought not presume anything about what a person would have wanted and should forgo any involvement in medical research generally and xenografting in particular on the grounds that this is what is demanded out of respect for the person he or she once was.

Severely retarded children and those born with devastating conditions such as anencephaly have never had the capacities and abilities that confer a greater moral standing on humans as compared with animals. Should they be used as the first donors and recipients in xenografting research instead of primates?

The reason they should not has nothing to do with the properties, capacities, and abilities of children or infants who lack and have always lacked significant degrees of intellectual and cognitive function. The reason they should not be used is because of the impact using them would have upon other human beings, especially their parents and relatives. A severely retarded child can still be the object of much love, attention, and devotion from his or her parents. These feelings and the abilities and capacities that generate them are deserving of moral respect. Animals do not appear to be capable of such feelings.

If a human mother were to learn that her severely retarded son had been used in lethal xenografting research, she would mourn this fact for the rest of her days. A baboon, monkey, dog, or pig would not. The difference counts in terms of whether it is a monkey or a retarded human being who is selected as a subject in xenografting research. Relationships and the impact of action on others count in ethics; and since this is less true or not at all true for animals, a bright chimp does not have greater moral standing then a severely retarded young boy, even if their intrinsic capacities are such that the chimp can do more than the boy.

It may be that parents would want to volunteer their child's organ or tissue for research or that they might wish to have their baby with anencephaly serve as the first recipient of an animal organ or tissue. I have argued that it may be morally permissible and even obligatory to respect such wishes. But the key moral point is that whatever public policies are created to govern our actions toward severely retarded children or babies born with most of their brains missing, these are policies that are meant to be respectful of the sensibilities and interests of other human beings. They do not find their source in some inherent property of the anencephalic infant. The assessment of the morals of how we treat each other and animals does not hinge simply on the properties that each possess. Relationships must enter into the equation as well, and when they do the balance begins to tip toward human rather than animal interests when there is a conflict. The moral worth and standing of the weak, the impaired, the unborn, and the injured is grounded not only in what they can do but what others feel for them in terms of respect, love, and concern.

If animals are to be used, then what sorts of guidelines should animal care and use committees or other review bodies follow in reviewing basic research proposals? These committees must ensure that basic research is designed in such a fashion as to minimize the need for animal subjects while maximizing the opportunity to obtain generalizable knowledge. They must also ensure that the animals used are kept in optimal conditions and are sacrificed humanely and without pain.

Perhaps the most difficult question arising when sufficient data has been obtained to make clinical trials plausible is who ought to be the first subjects in clinical xenografting trials. The Baby Fae infant heart baboon transplant case involved an infant because the researchers felt that the scarcity of organs for infants born with congenital defects was so great that morality demanded that infants be the initial subjects selected. Many argued that this choice was mistaken, since at the level of initial clinical trials it is morally wrong to use infants, children, or other human beings incapable of giving informed consent to their participation (Caplan, 1985).

If it is true that clinical trials involving xenografting should avoid the initial use of infants, children, and adults who lack the capacity for consent, then who ought to go first? Perhaps the first recipients should be adults who would not otherwise be eligible for transplants under existing exclusion criteria, the imminently dying, terminally ill volunteers who agree to serve, those who are brain dead, or those needing a second or third transplant when scarcity and prognosis would make it most unlikely they would receive another human organ or tissue.

Similarly, for clinical trials the question arises as to which type of organ or tissue ought to be the subject of initial research efforts? Those for which the scarcity of human organs and tissues is greatest or those for whom alternatives to animals organs seem the least promising? A strong case can be made that the selection of an organ or tissue to xenograft should be guided by the scarcity of human organs and tissues as well as the results achieved in animal to animal xenografting during basic research.

When clinical trials are designed for human subjects, those undertaking the research must have the qualifications and the background to make it likely that they will generate reliable and replicable results that are quickly made available in the literature. While the use of primates and human beings in research may be morally justified, it is ethical only when the research is designed and conducted in circumstances most likely to maximize the chance of creating valuable knowledge in the service of an important goal (IOM, 1996).

Those who will be recruited for clinical trials have the right to know the risks and benefits of the research as they can best be inferred from animal and any other relevant studies. They should also know how many subjects will be used before the end point of this phase of research is reached. The measures taken for coping with any psychological issues raised by the use of animal organs for subjects must be presented. Subjects should also be told about the steps that have been taken to ensure their privacy and confidentiality to the extent they wish to have them preserved. It is of special importance, given the high odds of failure in the initial phase of xenografting on human subjects, that procedures be in place for ending the experiment if the subject wishes to withdraw from the research.

ANIMAL ISSUES

Perhaps the most obvious moral problem that arises if xenografting proves to be a viable source of organs and tissue for transplantation is whether prospective recipients would be able to accept animal parts when in need of transplants. Some might feel that it is unnatural to do so. Naturalness, however, is very much a function of familiarity. And the prospect of death also has a powerful ability to shape a person's willingness to adapt to the new and "unnatural."

One hundred years ago, surgery seemed unnatural. For a surgeon to touch a beating heart was considered out of the question. But as the efficacy of surgery and surgery upon the heart were shown, the unnaturalness of these interventions was overtaken by the enthusiasm doctors and patients had for their impact on survival and health. People may require support and counseling when faced with the option of xenografting, but my hunch is that faced with death and no other choices, nearly all will accept a transplant from a pig or genetically altered cow or goat and decide to deal with the naturalness issue later.

What about systematically raising and killing animals for transplant on a large scale? Is it moral to systematically farm and kill animals for spare parts for humans? Is it right to systematically farm and kill animals for spare parts for other animals, say companion animals such as dogs and cats who might survive with transplants from pigs or sheep?

The systematic farming of animals for organs is a practice that strikes many as morally repugnant. But animals that are specially bred for transplant harvesting will be among the healthiest and happiest creatures on the globe. Mistreatment and poor health are unlikely for such animals, since those who receive their organs will want assurances that they are healthy and viable as can be.

Moreover, killing the animals in any way that causes stress or suffering would be unacceptable, not only from humane decency but also because stress may cause harm to the animals. Suffering and mishandling may be common in some areas of meat and poultry production, but they would have no role in organ farming. Liability for a flawed organ that can be traced to mistreatment of the animal on the part of a breeder or shipper would be enormous.

Despite all the attention paid to primates in current research, they are not going to be used on a large scale or farmed. If xenografting works, primate farming is not feasible because of difficulties in breeding, small brood sizes, and size mismatch problems between primate parts and people parts. When the issue is farming and harvesting, the animals are going to have to be of a physical scale such that their organs are close in size to those of humans—probably pigs, sheep, or cows.

Is it right to kill thousands of pigs assuming harvesting their organs would mean that there would be a good chance of saving an equivalent number of human lives? Pigs are relatively intelligent creatures. Pigs have the capacity for some thought and perhaps primitive intentionality. It must be conceded that they can be hurt, stressed, and made to suffer. These facts count in terms of the moral treatment of pigs, but while telling as factors that ought shape the use of pigs for food, they are not definitive barriers to the use of pigs to save lives.

Humans have, or at least have the potential if they are children, to do more than feel pain or experience pleasure. They experience more than animals do because they exist in social relationships with others that confer meaning and significance upon even the most deformed, disabled, or damaged member of this species. Given the choice between the need to kill a pig and the need to kill a child, the choice seems obvious, even if the child is retarded, mentally ill, or a newborn without consciousness. Why? Because the death of the child not only means the loss of the potential that the child might have had but also has an adverse impact on the child's relatives and family and an even wider negative impact on human beings who assign value, if only symbolic, to the rules and customs that protect their own lives and those of their children. Pigs do not construct such systems and do not live in accordance with such symbols, and these facts are morally relevant when life hangs in the balance.

Animals have many traits that are deserving of moral consideration and respect. But to treat them as equals in matters of life and death ignores what differentiates them from us. While to some extent the degree of difference is a matter of empirical fact, it is also true that the aim or reason for killing either animals or people makes a difference in the moral assessment of either. Systematically raising and killing millions of pigs for breakfast may make no moral sense. Systematically breeding thousands of genetically altered pigs to save human lives makes a great deal of moral sense.

eleven

Am I My Brother's Keeper? Ethics and the Use of Living Donors

The Use of Living Donors

MANY OBSERVERS BELIEVE THAT THE MOST promising option for increasing the supply of organs available for transplantation in the near future is increasing the number of living donors (Elick et al., 1990; Evans, 1989; Rapaport, 1986; Smith et al., 1986; Spital, 1991; Spital and Spital, 1985, 1988). A number of transplant programs in the United States and other nations have either expanded their use of living donors or are contemplating doing so.

The pressure to consider live donation often arises from the transplant candidate's family members and friends, who, wishing to help, volunteer to donate (Spital and Spital, 1985). In some nations the use of living persons is seen as ethically acceptable, particularly when there are inadequate resources for obtaining cadaver organs or religious and cultural prohibitions against cadaveric procurement (Johny et al., 1990).

Using living donors not only expands the potential pool of prospective organ donors but offers additional technical advantages. Transplants using organs from living donors can be scheduled in advance, thereby diminishing the emergency nature of transplant surgery characteristic of transplants in which cadaver organs are used. The ability to schedule surgery may permit the optimal use of expensive hospital resources and personnel (Spital and Spital, 1988), thereby lowering the overall costs associated with organ transplants.

The use of live donors also permits transplant teams to monitor the health of prospective donors; eliminates the need for organ preservation, storage, and shipping; allows more time for the testing and screening of organs for infectious diseases; and provides an advantage to recipients in that the transplanted organ begins to function immediately (Squifflet et al., 1990). Live donation may even make it possible to "pretreat" both donors and recipients in various ways that may increase the chances of successful transplants (Squifflet et al., 1990).

There are obvious limits on which organs can safely be removed from living persons. While a heart cannot be removed, duplicate organs such as the kidney and lung may be removed without impairing the donor. The risks to donors from surgery, while real, appear to be extremely small (Smith et al., 1986; Johny et al., 1990; Squifflet et al., 1990). Some organs, such as the liver and pancreas, will regenerate, permitting removal of pieces or segments from living donors. The risks to donors associated with the removal of lobes or segments of solid organs from living persons are not fully understood, but they appear to be small (Singer et al., 1989; Strong et al., 1990)

Experience with the efficacy of pancreas and liver transplantation using segments taken from living donors is preliminary but encouraging. The use of lobes of lung from living donors remains highly experimental. The best available data on efficacy of living organ donation involves kidneys. Outcomes in terms of graft and patient survival are as good or even slightly better than the rates of success achieved with cadaver donors (Elick et al., 1990; Spital and Spital, 1988).

Ethical Objections to Living Donation

Many within medicine believe that the practice of using living donors is unethical. Causing harm to a person solely to benefit another seems a violation of one of the core principles of medical ethics—do no harm. Others will only tolerate the practice as "transitional," something to be "gradually replaced" by some other option (Conference of European Health Ministers, 1987; Hamburger and Crosnier, 1968; McCormick, 1978; Kreis, 1985; Starzl, 1985; Council of Europe, 1996).

Some European nations, while allowing living donations, view the practice as ethically dubious (Conference of European Health Ministers, 1987; Evans, 1989; Sells and Wing, 1989; Swedish Committee on Transplantation, 1989; Squifflet et al., 1990). Whereas about a third of all kidneys transplanted in the United States come from living donors (Smith et al., 1986), the percentage of such donors in some European nations has been and remains far lower (Sells and Wing, 1989). In some nations, such as France, increases in cadaver organ donation have led to a proportional decrease in the use of live donors, which indicates that there is grave moral uncertainty about the practice (Caplan, 1992a).

Those opposed to the practice of using living human beings are especially worried about the morality of imposing risks and harms on those who provide organs or parts of organs. There is also concern about the ability of those who donate to give truly free and voluntary consent. Without voluntary consent, the use of living persons is taking not giving, battery not altruism.

RISKS AND HARMS

There are two distinct schools of thought about the morality of asking donors to face grave risks, albeit with a low probability of occurrence, in order to obtain an organ or part of an organ for someone in need of a transplant. Some, who might be termed "absolutists," claim that the imposition of serious risk by physicians upon a person for any non-therapeutic purpose is immoral (Ramsey, 1970). Imposing mortal risk violates the core moral precept against doing harm, nonmaleficence, which is seen to strongly bind physicians.

Others, who might be termed "proportionalists," object to living donation only if the imposition of harm or risk seems disproportionate to the benefit that will likely be attained (Bleich, 1993; Hamburger and Crosnier, 1968; McCormick, 1978; Starzl, 1985). Small risks might be acceptable in the service of near-certain benefits, but great risks for unknown benefits would not be. The test of the morality of imposing risk or harm is proportionality: are the benefits so certain and of a kind that they manifestly outweigh the risks of harm?

CONSENT

Others, less worried about the imposition or assumption of risk, believe individuals should be free to make decisions about how much risk and what sorts of risk they wish to face (Spital and Spital, 1985, 1988).

Instead, there is concern that it is simply not possible for a living donor to give true, voluntary informed consent to donation (Kreis, 1985; Starzl, 1985). The reasons why some feel valid consent in the context of live donation is compromised and might even be impossible fall into three categories: information, competency and coercion.

Information

Valid consent cannot be given to live donation without an individual's having an objective understanding of the risks and hazards involved. In order to provide valid consent, a person must have all relevant information and the opportunity to reflect upon and ask questions about the information from those who will provide objective answers.

Transplant centers and other transplant personnel may face problems in providing "objective" information to prospective donors because those involved in seeking donors have an inherent conflict of interest (Singer et al., 1989). They cannot advocate for the best interest of patients who need transplants and simultaneously protect the best interests of prospective donors. Those involved in innovative forms of live donation may be so eager to proceed that their enthusiasm may color the extent or kind of information made available to prospective donors. This is especially so when the same physician or health care team is treating both the prospective donor and the would-be recipient.

Competency

Approaching persons with impaired or absent competency in live donations raises problems for consent. Many persons have criticized the use of children, the retarded, and the mentally ill as live donors on the grounds that they lack the ability to consent to donation (Hamburger and Crosnier, 1968). Some nations prohibit using people under the age of eighteen as living donors of either organs or tissues on the grounds that they lack the ability to give informed consent. In the United States, most state courts have held that children and the mentally retarded cannot be compelled to donate to siblings or family members even when they are the only known source of potentially life-saving tissues or organs (Bleich, 1993).

Coercion

Finally, many critics of live donation worry that the environment in which live donation takes place makes it impossible for anyone to give free and voluntary consent. Family members will ordinarily feel extraordinary pressures to "volunteer." The realization that one could be blamed for the failure to help a spouse, a sibling, or a child may be so frightening that potential donors see themselves as having no choice. If a transplant fails when a spouse or family member has acted as the donor, other family members may feel overwhelmed by the pressure to "volunteer" as donors (Majeske, Parker, and Frader, 1996).

Even nonfamily members may feel they have no option but to indicate their willingness to donate organs or tissues. A stranger may feel coerced into volunteering when the ability to find other possible donors is limited by time or other factors (Singer et al., 1989).

Risk and Biological Relationships

The arguments against the use of living donors, whether based on moral concerns about the imposition of risks and harms or on the dubious prospects for informed consent, are frequently couched in all-or-none terms. Live donation is either ethically permissible or forbidden. Painting with this broad a brush is unfortunate, since the objections to the practice of living donation may not have equal force in all cases of live donation. The nature of biological and emotional ties that may or may not exist between donors and recipients may play a crucial role in deciding whether concerns about risks and the possibility of valid consent are such as to make live donation immoral.

Some believe that risks can never be imposed unless the aim of medical intervention is therapy for the person bearing the risks. They will not accept the imposition of risk even with consent as moral (Ramsey, 1970; Starzl, 1985). Others would permit the imposition of risk to benefit another if the risk is proportionate to the intended benefit.

But the presence or absence of risk and benefit is not the entire story in thinking about the ethics of consent to organ donation. In order to assess proportionality, it is necessary to know the nature of the biological relationships that exist between the prospective donor and recipient.

Some forms of live donation involve taking organs or tissues from a donor who is biologically related to the potential recipient. There is significant controversy about the exact importance of biological differences between donor and recipient for the success of transplants. But for some forms of transplantation, biology makes a difference in the probability of achieving success.

Related donors are those persons who have a close biological relationship, in terms of blood and antigen types, with someone requiring an organ. Similarities in blood and antigen types result from familial inheritance or, far less often, chance genetic similarities. Identical twins are the only persons who have a complete coincidence of biological identity and therefore the best odds of success in transplantation.

Biologically unrelated donors can also be used for transplantation. Powerful immunosuppresive drugs make it possible to attempt transplants between persons known to have significant biological differences. But these drugs, such as Cyclosporin and FK 506, carry other risks of harm for recipients. Many transplant surgeons are much more comfortable about the chances of success of a transplant when the donor is biologically related to the recipient.

The assessment of how much risk and how much harm can reasonably be offered to a prospective living donor is inevitably a function of the predicted likelihood that the transplant will succeed. The chance of producing a benefit usually hinges on the degree of biological similarity that exists between donor and recipient. Those willing to accept proportionality will consider the morality of undertaking live donation to be greater when there is a biological relationship between donor and recipient and more dubious when there is no biological tie.

Harms and Emotional Relationships

Those who object to live donation due to a lack of proper proportionality or concerns regarding consent face another problem. There is no universal magic number or ratio such that proportionality can be shown to be satisfied. The assessment of what is an acceptable risk will vary according to the identity of the person who is being asked to bear that risk.

Nor is it possible in the real world to determine the validity of consent without some attention to the specific characteristics and relationships that apply to prospective donors. The donor may be emotionally related to the intended recipient, either because they are family members or through other emotional ties. Emotional relationships may be positive or negative. Whichever they are, they have particular relevance for understanding the validity of consent.

The only way to assess worries about risk and consent is to examine the kinds of relationships that might obtain between donor and recipient. Most biologically unrelated donors have some existing emotional relationship with the prospective recipient, for example in-law, spouse, ex-spouse, friend, adoptive parent, lover, or co-worker. It is also possible for a potential donor to be biologically related to a prospective recipient but to have no emotional ties with the person in need. This would be true, for instance, of a man who had donated sperm to be used for artificial insemination but had played no parenting role whatsoever toward the children created using his sperm, or for a man whose sperm was used posthumously to create a child. It is also possible, if exceedingly rare, for complete strangers to be closely related in terms of blood and tissue type.

Possible Relationships among Living Donors and Recipients

	Biologically Related (BR)	Not Biologically Related (NBR)
Emotionally Related (ER)	Sibling, aunt/uncle, parent (BER)	Spouse, lover, stepchild, foster parent, surrogate mother (NBER)
Not Emotionally Related (NER)	Divorced and remarried parent; anonymous sperm/egg donor; sibling separated at birth; birth parent of adopted child; postmortem conception via frozen sperm (BNER)	Stranger, distant cousin by marriage (NBNER)

As the table illustrates, a wide variety of ties, both biological and emotional, may exist between potential live donors and recipients. Biologically related prospective donors may lose their emotional ties with prospective recipients, while biologically unrelated prospective donors may have powerful preexisting emotional bonds with prospective recipients.

Emotional relationships can develop if contact is permitted between a prospective living donor and a recipient. In this analysis, however, the terms "emotionally related" and "not related" refer only to preexisting ties or the lack thereof between prospective donors and potential recipients.

The taxonomy makes it clear that live donation is not readily evaluated on moral grounds as an all-or-nothing practice. The ethical issues raised by the practice vary, depending upon whether the donor is biologically and emotionally related (BER), biologically but not emotionally related (BNER), not biologically related but emotionally related (NBER), or neither biologically nor emotionally related (NBNER) to the would-be recipient. The complicated stew of relationships that must be taken into account in assessing the morality of using a living person as a source of organs or tissues is described in the table.

The Imposition of Risk upon Donors

The availability of a taxonomy showing the range of relationships that can and do exist in the domain of live donors helps to reveal important facts about the morality of imposing risk and harm. A position that sees any imposition of risk except for purposes of therapeutic benefit to the person assuming the risk as immoral (Ramsey, 1970) is simply inconsistent with the moral roles of either spouse or parent. Parents and spouses are expected and obligated, both in the law and in moral theory, to assume certain risks and bear harms for the sole purpose of providing benefits to their children or mates (see Donaldson, 1993, especially 28–34, and Smith, 1993). Those who adhere to a position that absolutely prohibits the nonegoistic imposition or assumption of risk must show why BER or NBER donors should be discouraged from assuming levels of risk they would feel obligated to assume and are required by law to bear in other contexts.

Those who believe that the risk can be imposed or assumed only in proportion to the likelihood of a beneficial outcome (McCormick, 1978; Starzl, 1985) must weigh both what is known about the relevance of biological relationships for the success of a particular form of transplant and the relationship that exists among donor and recipient. What might be viewed as a reasonable assumption of risk between a BER donor and recipient, for example a mother providing a lobe of a liver or lung to her daughter, might not be seen as proportionate in a situation in which a complete stranger, who is not of a similar tissue and blood type, is asked to serve as the source of a lobe of an organ for a dying child. Proportionality cannot be assessed without paying attention to the responsibilities and duties that adhere in the relationships and bonds between prospective donors and recipients. A mother who is not allowed to donate to her child may suffer not only because her child may die but also because she feels she is not being allowed to be a good mother.

Harm and Informed Consent

Informed consent depends upon the ability of a person to comprehend information, understand the available options, make a choice without penalty, have adequate time and an environment conducive to deliberation, and be able to withdraw at any time (President's Commission, 1983; Faden and Beauchamp, 1986). If these conditions are sound, there would appear to be reasons for concern about the ability of some live donors to give valid informed consent.

There are some who believe that no imposition of risk is moral without voluntary, explicit, informed consent. And there are many potential donors who lack the capacity for consent. These include the mentally ill, those who are severely retarded, the demented elderly, children, those in permanent comas, fetuses, and perhaps prisoners and other institutionalized persons. Those holding this view will under any circumstances oppose the use of living donors who are incapable of consent. Incompetent persons can serve as sources but not as donors.

Depending on the nature of the biological and emotional relationships that exist, however, the inability to consent may not provide an absolute barrier to live donation. This has been the position of a number of U.S. courts that have approved the procurement of a kidney from a minor child (*Strunk v. Strunk,* 1969; *Hart v. Brown,* 1972) with parental consent and from a severely retarded boy (*Little v. Little,* 1979) on the grounds that the nature of the biological and emotional relationships that existed between the donor and the prospective recipient outweighed the inability of the donor to consent (see, however, *In re Richardson* [1973], a decision by the Court of Appeals of Louisiana, Fourth Circuit, for a strict absolutist position against any form of donation from a minor child).

It is possible that members of these groups could be used as living donors if another person acted as a surrogate or proxy decision maker. If proxies are permitted, they must make decisions based upon their view of the prospective donor's best interest.

The nature of the relationship between prospective donor and recipient may alter the perception of best interest that a proxy makes. A proxy may feel that BER and NBER donors have different interests in facing the risks inherent in donation than someone who is BNER or NBNER. For example, a young boy who is retarded may not understand the risks of donating a segment of his pancreas to his brother. However, the proxy may feel that it is still in the boy's interest to donate if there is a strong bond between the brothers.

Even when a potential donor is indisputably competent, the nature of the emotional relationship that exists with a potential recipient may still alter the ability to give informed consent to donation. BER and NBER donors may find it impossible to give their consent freely, either because they feel coerced by subtle but nonetheless real pressure from other family members or simply by the nature of the obligations that they see as defining their relationship (Smith, 1986) to the person in need. Oddly, those who have no emotional ties to prospective recipients may sometimes be in a better position to satisfy concerns about consent than are those persons who have emotional ties to prospective recipients.

If consent is to be valid, then those giving it must feel free to say no. This is especially true in situations where emotional ties create pressures that would render the relationship impossible in the future were the prospective donor to refuse. In such situations, those seeking consent must be willing to provide a "cover story" or some form of "medical excuse" for prospective donors who wish to refuse or withdraw their consent. Those unwilling to make it possible for BER and NBER donors to choose without penalty might be wise to search only among BNER and NBNER donors.

Finally, the selection of proxies in situations where the donor is manifestly not competent must be sensitive to the emotional tie between the proxy and both the prospective donor and the potential recipient. Nowhere is this more evident than in situations where a couple conceives a child in the hope of finding a tissue or an organ donor. Proxies must be able to weigh the best interest of the incompetent and vulnerable donor. It might be wise to insist upon third-party review for any situation in which an incompetent person is to be used as a donor on the basis of a proxy consent.

Is Live Donation an Ethically Acceptable Option?

None of the objections raised against the use of living persons as the source of organs for transplants provides adequate grounds for a complete prohibition of the practice. Those who believe that it is wrong for physicians to impose harm or risks if the person bearing the harm or risk will not benefit from the intervention have not made a persuasive case. Some emotional relationships require the bearing of risks. The wide and complex range of donor-recipient relationships means that moral matters regarding the use of living donors are too complicated to capture under a simple "yes" or "no" framework. Incompetent donors pose special problems. Yet even for this group of prospective donors, the nature of emotional and biological ties to prospective recipients may allow their use as living donors in some circumstances using proxies to provide consent.

There are other persons, manifestly competent, whose emotional relationship with the prospective recipient nonetheless calls into question their ability to provide consent. Those who see live donation as morally justified only when consent is freely given may have to argue for the use of persons who are less than ideally suited biologically but who are well suited emotionally in order to ensure that donation is preceded by a valid consent.

Perhaps the greatest source of moral unease about live donation is that it will lead inevitably to the creation of a commercial market in organs. This fear has motivated most of the legislative and regulatory action undertaken with respect to live donation (Council of the Transplantation Society, 1985; Swedish Committee on Transplantation, 1989; Caplan, 1992a). Certainly moral revulsion at the prospect of a market in human organs must be taken seriously by anyone advocating live donation. In actuality, a wide variety of public policies are compatible with live donation. The strategies of using free markets, presumed consent, required request, and pure voluntarism, policies familiar in the debates about cadaver donation (see chapter 9), all have potential application to live donation.

It is almost always presumed in current discussions of live donation that regardless of emotional or biological ties, those who might serve as living donors of organs or parts of organs would act under a public policy framework of altruistic voluntarism. Health professionals or families need not be required to pursue the option of live donation or even to make inquiries about donation to possible donors. This situation could be changed.

A policy closely akin to that which exists in the United States regarding required requests for cadaver donation (Caplan, 1992a) could be implemented. Legislation could be enacted requiring that the option of donation be presented to all potential living donors. Transplant centers, procurement organizations, and patients and their families could be required to pursue the option of securing a living donor. Or a required request policy might be limited to making requests only of those persons known to be emotionally related to a person seeking an organ. The desire to respect the principle of proportionality might lead to a policy of required request aimed only at those known to be biologically related to the prospective recipient.

A society could decide to institute presumed-consent policies toward living donation similar to those that prevail in European nations such as France, Belgium, and Austria and in many states governing the procurement of corneas and tissues from unclaimed bodies under the control of coroners or medical examiners. Those known to be possible sources of organs, regardless of their emotional and perhaps even biological relationships, would have to donate (strong presumed consent) or at least bear the burden of proof as to why they should not (weak presumed consent). The attempt in 1990 to persuade an Illinois court to compel bone marrow donation from a minor for a nonemotionally related half-sibling against the objection of a parent is a concrete illustration of the problems a presumed-consent policy would actually face. The Illinois Supreme Court ruled in Bosze, 141 Ill.2d 473 at 484, that there was no basis for presuming that the minor twins had developed any sort of values or judgments and ruled against a mother's impassioned request to tissue type the twins to see if they might be suitable marrow donors.

Finally, a society might decide to permit one of a variety of forms of free market in the domain of live donation. Any living donor, regardless of biological or emotional ties, could be allowed to offer organs in return for compensation, such as cash, discounts on health or life insurance, guarantees of burial costs, and free medical care. Those who actually make organs available might receive priority with respect to access to transplants or other forms of medical care. Singapore has adopted something close to this policy (Teo, 1991).

A society may find it morally repugnant to allow the sale of organs between sources and recipients with certain emotional or biological ties (Kearney and Caplan, 1992). It may seem repugnant to allow a brother to sell his kidney to his sister. Market approaches are morally suspect (chapter 9). But if they are to be allowed, it is hard to see on what basis restrictions on sale could be imposed or enforced.

Expanding the use of living donors may well be the most feasible option for quickly reducing the gap between the supply of and the demand for transplantable organs. The practice of using living related donors is still in its infancy. There is a great deal of ethical disquiet about the idea of removing organs or parts of organs from persons with the sole goal of benefiting others. Thus the policy options described here have not been pursued with any particular zeal.

Donation by living persons who can choose to do so is not ethically wrong, at least in some situations, and it is clearly morally right and obligatory in a few situations, as when a parent can provide bone marrow to a child in need. Oddly, those involved in donation who have close emotional ties or are bound by love may be obligated to donate but less able to choose to do so. Only strangers can truly choose to undertake some risks even if they are under little or no obligation to choose to do so. Those who have no emotional ties to those in need but have the capacity to understand the risks involved in giving an organ ought to be permitted to do so on the condition that they undergo a careful assessment of their competency. If some of the ethical obstacles to the use of living donors are removed, it is vital that a debate commence as to the merits of the policy options that living donation presents in order to establish which are likely to provide benefits to those in need while minimizing risks and harms for those who choose to help them.

PART FOUR

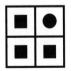

HEALTH POLICY

twelve

Dead as a Doornail

HAS THE TIME COME TO RETHINK THE definition of death in the United States? Many experts in medicine, ethics, and the law think so. But is the American public interested in a reexamination of how death is defined? That is far from certain. And even if the American people were willing to listen to new ideas about the definition of death, would the price of stirring this particular pot be too much to pay? Yes—this is a pot that should not be brought to a conceptual boil; the price is not worth paying.

One reason for pessimism about reopening a discussion of how best to define death is the absolute lack of consensus about what a new definition ought to be. The differences of opinion are so great that an effort to shift public opinion as well as actual practice in medicine and the law would create much more harm than benefit.

Some would argue that consensus is not the point. Or, rather, the absence of consensus is exactly the point. If disagreements exist about the nature of death, then public opinion, medical practice, and the law must reflect this fact.

But it is not at all clear that in matters of life and death the only response a pluralistic society should offer in the face of dissent is to respect, accept, and formalize different points of view. The desire to monkey with a fundamental concept, such as death most certainly is, has to be weighed against society's need for stability and clarity about when life is over. The best way to respect differences of opinion about the nature of death in a pluralistic society may well be to avoid rocking a boat that might well capsize.

What does the public think about the need to redefine death? Although I have spent a lot of time arguing that bioethics ought to be done in public (Caplan, 1992a) and engaged in this activity myself (Caplan, 1995a), I have little understanding of the level of public confidence in the prevailing definition of death. Nor can I discern what definition commands the greatest popular support.

These inabilities are not peculiar to me. There is little empirical evidence about public attitudes and beliefs about death or the definition of death in the United States or anywhere else. Prescribing the nature of the relationship between expertise and public policy with respect to death is difficult. It is especially so when the experts do not agree about what death is and when it is not clear that the public follows their disagreements or believes there is any reason to care about them.

Worse still from the point of view of trying to decide whether the time has come to revisit the definition of death, it is hard to know how much philosophical nuance and scientific ambiguity the public will put up with when it comes to death. Experts may think *death* is an ambiguous term, about which people of good will can disagree. Laymen may well think the experts are all nuts if they cannot agree on what death is.

Some experts warn that our society has already mucked around with the definition of death quite enough and that it is dangerous to even talk about the subject in public. Others argue that it was a mistake to try to define death by consensus in the first place. It was wrong to try to define death by committee at Harvard roughly thirty years ago, remained wrong fifteen years later in Washington when a presidential commission went to bat, and is not something that wrangling among members of another committee, blue-ribbon panel, or commission would speed toward a resolution today. The effort to redefine or refine definitions by committee and commission ought, some say, to cease.

Still other experts seem certain that the need for revisiting the subject of defining death by committee, commission, or other public body is obvious and has never been more pressing (Gervais, 1986; Emanuel, 1995; Singer, 1995; Veatch, 1993). Some believe (Halevy and Brody, 1993; Truog, 1997) that the United States had better rush to revisit the definitions and diagnostic tests already promulgated in existing public policy and clinical practice lest the current law continue to trample on the religious and philosophic freedoms of U.S. citizens. It is not right to ask those who see death differently from the way doctors now do to live under the yoke of only two standards of death (cardiopulmonary or total brain) unless they are lucky enough to live in New Jersey, where they may avail themselves of merely one if they so choose, or in the State of New York, where health care providers are enjoined to be reasonably accommodating to individual preferences about the definition of death. However, the case for accommodation is somewhat weakened by the spectacle of seeing persons pronounced dead twice, as happened to a newborn girl, Mariah Scoon, in New York City who was pronounced dead at one hospital only to be transferred and pronounced dead yet again a month later (Caplan, 1996c).

Other problems favoring a revisiting of existing legal and medical standards include the fact that people, especially young children, are sometimes called dead inconsistently; the failure to obtain organs for transplants because of obsession with imposing arbitrary standards of death; the blatant waste from failure to cut the costs of caring for certain categories of patients who cannot benefit because they are basically dead; and the risk of undertreatment for those who would wish it or whose families wish it even when others might say death has come (Brini, 1996; Caplan, 1995a, 1996b, c).

Despite a lack of unanimity among experts about what death is and about what this diversity of opinion means for public policy and despite the lack of any solid evidence as to what the public thinks about these matters, the issue still arises as to whether the time is ripe for trying to refine the definition of death in the United States. It isn't.

The arguments in favor of change rely on three claims: There is a better way of defining death. There is sufficient difference of opinion about the definition of death that a single definition ought not be imposed on all. And there is no essential feature characteristic of death, so any attempt at a definition is doomed.

The most persuasive reason for change is the view that the existing definition of death is inaccurate. There is, however, no agreement about the nature of the inaccuracy. Depending on whom you listen to, the prevailing definition of death—permanent loss of cardiorespiratory function or total and irreversible loss of all brain function—is either too narrow or too broad.

Some argue brain death should be replaced by a definition that permits the equation of death with the cessation of something less than all brain function. It is thinking and consciousness that count for any meaningful conception of life. Therefore death should mean complete cortical death, "higher" brain death, or the irreversible loss of those brain functions involved in consciousness (Gervais, 1986; Wikler, 1988; Veatch, 1993).

A few worry that the methods for ascertaining brain or cardiac death are not up-to-date. New technology such as highly sensitive blood-flow measurement techniques, PET scans, and brain metabolism tests could merit change if not in the definition then certainly in the tests used to determine death. It might raise the cost of dying a great deal, but more precision is possible.

Others argue that the end of all vital signs, whether maintained artificially or not, is crucial to some Americans in order that death be pronounced. While not endorsing this vitalistic view, many believe that the cultural, religious, or ethnic beliefs of the arguably deceased and his or her close family, kin, partner, or religious leader ought to set the bar over which the Grim Reaper must be required to jump before death is pronounced (Post, 1995). If some want to say there is no death until no signs of life or biological activity can be discerned, who is to say they are wrong? If people believe in vitalism, then it should be reflected in law and medical practice.

The fact is that the mere existence of a disagreement about what is sufficient to say that death has come is enough to refute those who want to shift the definition to a broader or a narrower place. To some extent the definition of death is arbitrary. More technology, repeated testing, could always be done to confirm the diagnosis. And whether self-awareness, the capacity to feel pain, or the ability to reason is requisite for meaningful or worthwhile life, a persuasive case has not been made that its absence is to be equated, or must be equated, with death. A human being who is permanently unconscious or who has been born without a brain may well lack the cognitive powers necessary to be a person in the legal sense of that term. But to say that unconscious or severely demented persons are dead is to stretch the definition of death so far as to make it unlikely that many will see the need.

A further problem with shifting to definitions of death that rely either on more technical measurements of brain activity or measurements of only some parts of the brain is that the public, the press, even many in health care have had a hard time absorbing the concept of brain death. The prospects for cementing public trust in a new standard of death when a twenty-year effort to advance understanding of brain death has sowed so much confusion and misunderstanding are neither inspiring nor rosy.

Then it might be argued that those who equate death with the permanent absence of mentation or the absence of self-awareness should be free to live their lives by this standard. But then the case for redefining death turns on the need for respecting differences of opinion. If some Americans, for religious, cultural, metaphysical, or personal reasons, dissent from the mainstream definition of death, does not a liberal democratic society have an obligation to respect their right to call themselves dead however it pleases them to do so?

An overarching reason for doing nothing in the face of disquiet on the part of some about the way death is defined is that the political cost of reopening the discussion would be staggering. The politics of death has historically been a mess in this country. There is no reason to presume it will be different if this can of worms is reopened any time soon.

There are very powerful interest groups who desire no change in the definition at the present time. These include right-to-life groups, disability groups, and leaders in organized religion. Their concerns about changing the definition of death were on display in the heated negative response that greeted the decision of the American Medical Association's Ethics and Judicial Council to endorse the use of anencephalic infants as donors of vital organs (Anonymous, 1995). Right-to-life groups and some religious organizations fear that opening up a discussion of redefining death will open the door to active, involuntary euthanasia of the severely retarded, the demented, and the comatose, and active euthanasia for these persons is such a powerfully charged issue that any effort to engage in a public debate about the definition of death is doomed. When powerful interest groups are willing to go to the mat to oppose a change on an issue that has no significant advocacy constituency, the prospects for change are nil and the cost of agitating for change is great.

The irony of having existing standards of whole brain death used as a shield to protect the interests of the comatose and of newborn disabled infants should not be lost. The major opposition to brain death came from those in religious and right-to-life circles, many of the same people and groups who are now most fervent in demanding no change in the whole brain death definition.

The fact is that some of those who argue for changes in the definition of death do so because they wish other changes to occur in public policy. Those who argue for a cortical or higher brain function standard often do so in the belief that persons in a permanent coma should be available for experiments or as organ and tissue donors. Some plump for an easier standard because they want to see less effort made by society in supplying resources to keep alive those who are permanently vegetative or anencephalic. The fact is that these other goals can be achieved without changing the boundaries of death.

Whatever the merits of the ideas, broadening the definition of organ donor or limiting efforts to keep those who are in a permanent vegetative state in intensive care units can be done without any shift in the definition of death. Indeed, moving the boundary of death as a tactic to achieve these other goals presents the impression that death is defined as a matter of convenience for organ procurement or as a matter of economic efficiency with respect to high-cost medical expenditures. Whatever else death is, it should not be a function of these sorts of considerations.

If there is no consensus among experts about the definition of death or no real political reason to impose one, then why not let more definitional flowers bloom? One state, New Jersey, altered its definition of death a few years ago to provide more choice and autonomy to individuals who might not subscribe to definitions that equate death with the absence of wavy lines on graph paper. No civil disorder resulted from the Garden State's decision to let death reside in the eye of the beholder. So those who tout change in the name of democracy and tolerance argue that New Jersey should be a model to us all, inspiring other jurisdictions to adopt pluralism in the definition of death.

The final reason for not clinging to the current definition of death is somewhat abstract. The existing definition rests on a fundamental philosophical error. The law now sees death as having a key or defining property. There is something fundamentally wrong with any "essentialist" conception of death, because death can be looked at in more ways than are ever dreamt of in any neurologist's universe. Actually, death is a process and not an event (Emanuel, 1995; Halevy and Brody, 1993). Any definition that uses essentialist language referring to a particular time or moment of death or any key neurological or physiological criterion is not, by definition, up to the task.

This line of argument is bolstered by the claim that not only is intolerance in this area immoral but the imposition of an arbitrary standard of death can harm people. If death is misdiagnosed, people may be hurt. Sometimes people are pronounced dead even though detectable brain activity is still present after the pronouncement (Halevy and Brody, 1996). Others are pronounced dead when the tests and measures used are known to be insufficient to establish its presence (Halevy and Brody, 1996). No wonder there is concern about the impact on the ability of the public to sleep soundly at night should discussions of revising brain death become loud and public.

A review of the arguments in favor of redefining death in public policy does not produce an impressive case. The main reason is that while there is much discussion of the alleged philosophical inadequacies of the existing definition of death as the total and irreversible cessation of either cardiac or brain function, there is nothing even close to a consensus about what banner the critics are willing to march under toward the state capitals. What is worse, it seems most unlikely that a mass political movement toward redefining death is likely to erupt, even under tender and thoughtful philosophical cultivation, given the current levels of mistrust of medicine (Caplan, 1996b). Since many Americans are worried about whether there will be enough money in their health plan to save their lives or if they will be turned away at the hospital door for want of insurance, the prospects for philosophical disquiet energizing a political movement to change how it is that medicine pronounces death are exceedingly slim. A climate of distrust is not propitious for opening the question of where doctors should redraw the line between who is dead and who is not.

The prospects for change are made even grimmer when one adds to the policy stew the argument that change is needed to open the door to a greater supply of organs for transplant. Talk of waiving the so-called "dead donor rule," which requires persons to be dead before vital organs are removed from their bodies, or expanding organ procurement to include those who are sort of dead, kind of dead, or close enough to dead is likely to fall on deaf ears—ears made particularly unreceptive by their perception that the system for allocating the supply of organs is not fair to begin with. Baseball star Mickey Mantle, TV star Larry Hagman, former Pennsylvania governor Robert Casey, and rock legend David Crosby may each have tried hard to promote organ donation after receiving transplants. But the belief that these gentlemen were accorded special access to transplants over others equally in need but less blessed by celebrity or wealth means there will be no interest in changing the line dividing life from death as a way to expand the pool of vital organs that might be transplanted to those who need them.

Perhaps the strongest case against trying to use philosophical acumen to pull public policy in the direction of either a broader view of death, a less essentialist conception, or one that permits a greater social good to be achieved by bumping the borders of mortality around a bit is that there is some evidence for thinking that such an effort is doomed to fail and would be dead on arrival in legislatures all around the United States. That evidence is the lack of trust in medicine brought on by shifts in the structure and financing of health care. Moving away from an essentialist conception of death, even toward a policy that is eclectic in its essentialism, will not happen when trust in those who pronounce death is low.

Nor should it. The definition of death is not simply about what is going on in the brain or the heart. It is also about what is going on between doctor and patient and between medicine and society. What is going on now is a revolution in the way care is delivered and paid for. Until the public feels it can put its faith in medicine once again, there is no chance they will trust those in white coats to redefine who it is that is dead.

thirteen

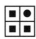

Sinners, Saints, and Access to Health Care

THE NOTION OF PERSONAL RESPONSIBILITY has played an important if not always explicit role in the allocation of resources for health care in the United States for many decades (Rosner, 1982; Adams, 1991), and the field of transplantation is no exception. A variety of criteria with presumed roots in personal responsibility, including mental status, patient compliance, criminal behavior, smoking, and the use of addictive drugs, have been used in making decisions about who receives access to scarce life-saving transplants (Levenson and Olbrish, 1993; Caplan, 1989d; Orentlicher, 1996). These decisions are often made, however, under the rubric of "psychosocial" contraindications to transplant. While many transplant teams, in their weekly meetings, think it appropriate to weigh into their allocation equation a history of felonious criminal conduct or the fact that someone is a prisoner, they are much more comfortable doing so under the rubric of "psychosocial suitability" than of "personal responsibility."

Transplant teams are not alone in trying to avoid any explicit reference to personal responsibility in their rationing decisions. Historically, physicians have tried to minimize the importance of responsibility in allocating health care resources. Doctors, nurses, and other health care professionals have recognized an ethical duty to treat those who require their services regardless of how they came to have their need.

In recent years, however, an increasing number of commentators have begun to call for a change in the traditional professional ethic requiring a duty to heal regardless of the character or conduct of the patient. Many authors believe that the time has come to invoke their notions of personal responsibility as morally relevant criteria for guiding allocation decisions in health care (Veatch, 1981; Menzel, 1990; Blank, 1988). Some believe physicians ought to take personal responsibility into account in making decisions at the bedside about who is eligible to receive treatment. Others argue that personal responsibility, while not a justifiable basis for excluding anyone from services, ought to play a role in physician decisions about what priority to assign to those competing for the same scarce resources. And more and more frequently, politicians, health policy analysts, and public health experts suggest that more weight should be given to personal responsibility in public policies aimed at reducing health care costs (Minnesota Health Reform Legislation, 1992). When President Bill Clinton launched his ill-fated health reform effort with a speech to Congress on September 23, 1993, he listed personal responsibility among the six values he said ought to guide the effort to reform the U.S. health care system.

The belief that certain behaviors ought to be grounds for disqualification when it comes to health care, at least of the expensive variety, is not only a matter of theory. Some primary care physicians will not accept people who smoke as their patients. Some have argued that those who abuse intravenous drugs ought to be denied access to surgery to repair heart valves damaged by endocarditis. Surgeons have assigned lower priority to smokers for access to bypass surgery. In some dialysis programs, those who are violent, abusive, or noncompliant are disqualified from treatment even if it means their certain death (Lowance, 1993). Many rehabilitation programs use psychosocial criteria, including assessment of compliance and motivation, as standard parts of their eligibility determinations in placing would-be patients on their waiting lists as well as in making decisions to terminate care (Haas et al., 1987). Most transplant programs turn away persons who are convicted criminals.

Notions of personal responsibility are beginning to play explicit roles in decisions about how governments allocate their overall budgets for health care. Many states and countries levy taxes on tobacco products and alcohol, at least in part because they think those who indulge in the use of such products ought to pay society for the health costs that accrue as a result of these unhealthy behaviors (Manning et al., 1991). Some governments permit insurers to charge higher premiums for groups or categories of persons who engage in harmful or risky personal behavior. Public health laws have been proposed or enacted that permit the prosecution

and incarceration of those whose irresponsible behavior has health consequences for others, such as the failure to stop taking narcotic drugs
during pregnancy, the failure to adequately control a vicious dog, or the
failure to make sure young children ride in car seats while traveling in
automobiles. The more that is learned about the connection between the
need for health care services and the high costs imposed by certain
behaviors on the rest of society (Manning et al., 1991), the more physicians and policymakers seem willing to use personal responsibility as an
appropriate criterion for allocating health care resources (Annas, 1985).

Organ transplantation occupies a key place in current debates about
the moral relevance of personal responsibility for the just allocation of
health care resources (Caplan, 1992a). Organs for transplant are scarce,
and rationing is both unavoidable and omnipresent. Transplants of solid
organs are expensive and require a variety of forms of public support and
subsidy. The stakes involved in transplantation are high, often amounting
to the difference between life and death, raising serious public concerns
about fairness and equity with respect to allocation policies. And since
transplantation depends upon community altruism for the supply of
cadaver organs, the public and its elected officials take an especially keen
interest in the equity of norms and values guiding allocation decisions in
the field of transplantation (Caplan, 1992a).

For many years those in the transplant community have treated alcoholism as a contraindication to various forms of organ transplantation.
This has been especially true with respect to liver transplants. In part this
was a result of the fact that initial reports on liver transplantation for
those who had alcohol-related liver cirrhosis suggested poor outcomes
and because of fears about recidivism with respect to alcohol abuse if a
transplant were performed (Atterbury, 1986; Lucey, 1993).

Recent reports indicate that patients with chronic liver disease due to
alcoholism who receive transplants do about as well in terms of survival
and psychological complications as those who require liver transplant for
other reasons (Lucey, 1993; Lucey and Beresford, 1992). Nor does there
appear to be a significant difference in the resources used by alcoholic and
nonalcoholic recipients. Short-term survival rates for those with both
alcoholic hepatitis and cirrhosis are not greatly different from rates for
those with only chronic cirrhosis. By controlling for the age of recipients,
some argue that liver transplantation could be accomplished as successfully in one group as in the other (Bonet et al., 1993).

What these findings do is force out into the open the moral issue of
whether personal responsibility should be taken into consideration in
allocating scarce and expensive resources. For if it is true that the cause

of liver failure in adults is far less predictive of a successful outcome than other factors such as age and co-morbidity, then it can only be values, not facts, that lead many programs to continue to exclude alcoholics from access to liver transplants.

There would appear to be three moral arguments for excluding alcoholics from access to liver transplants. The same arguments can be used to assign those who abuse liquor lower priority should there be other potential recipients who might be equally in need of a liver transplant.

It might be argued that those who bring harm upon themselves do not merit an investment of a large share of societal resources to repair that harm (Annas, 1985; Lucey and Beresford, 1992; Bonet et al., 1993). If a Mickey Mantle or a David Crosby destroys his liver as a result of drug or alcohol abuse, then he should not be entitled to a new one. Self-destruction is seen by many as its own reward, at least when it comes to booze. Few things can get the blood pressure of the average American up more than finding out that a celebrity alcoholic seems to have snuck to the front of the waiting list for a transplant.

Some contend that it is not past sin but future vice that ought to count against those in need of a liver transplant. Those who are at high risk of causing themselves harm again in the future ought be excluded from access to expensive medical interventions such as liver transplantation (Atterbury, 1986; Lucey, 1993; Lucey and Beresford, 1992; Orentlicher, 1996).

And there are those who maintain that it is unwise for the transplant field to permit access to transplants for those suffering from cirrhosis or hepatitis resulting from alcohol abuse because this population is of a size sufficient to exclude nearly all other patients suffering from liver failure. If alcohol abusers were to make up the overwhelming majority of those receiving liver transplants, public support for the transplant field would evaporate as a result of the stigma and opprobrium many citizens feel for those who abuse alcohol (Moss and Siegler, 1991).

None of these arguments is persuasive. While it might be viewed as unfair for society to invest large amounts of resources to repair harm resulting from lifestyle or personal behavior, there is no reason to single out alcohol abuse as especially worthy of punitive exclusion from important medical services. Put aside the question of whether alcoholism is a voluntarily chosen behavior (Lucey and Beresford, 1992; Fingarette, 1988) or a disease. Fairness requires that like cases be treated alike, so exclusionary policies in terms of access to expensive medical care would be in order for individuals who harm themselves as a result of participating in sports, riding horseback, failing to wear a seatbelt while driving or a helmet while biking, failing to obey speed limits, smoking, using too much aspirin, owning and using a firearm, being morbidly obese, working in environments that are dangerous or stressful, owning a large dog or a swimming pool, or living a sedentary life in front of the TV.

A more persuasive case can be made for excluding from access or assigning lower priority to those who require retransplantation, since giving someone a new organ that he or she will then simply proceed to damage does not make sense. But this is hardly the same as excluding alcoholics regardless of whether they are now sober or will try to be. The recidivism rates associated with liver transplantation are sufficiently low as to make fears of future abuse a weak predictor of successful transplant outcomes (Lucey, 1993; Lucey and Beresford, 1992; Cohen and Benjamin, 1991).

Most ironically of all, it may not be fair to exclude those who drink from consideration for a transplant if the primary source of donated livers are those who die as a result of their own alcohol abuse (Bonet et al., 1993). Presumably many of these people and their families would not want to exclude others who drink from consideration as candidates for receiving organs.

Finally, there may be truth to the argument that a field which serves only those who abuse alcohol risks alienating the general public. But many fields, such as psychiatry, psychology, oncology, infectious disease, and emergency medicine, must cope with the reality of stigma, fear, prejudice, and bias with respect to their patients. The proper response to the problem of stigma is not to exclude patients who might benefit from transplants but to educate the public about the importance of providing fair access to those in need and to call for the redoubling of efforts to find solutions to alcohol abuse (Cohen and Benjamin, 1991).

In the end, the data is not ambivalent. Those whose livers fail as a result of alcohol abuse can do about as well as others whose livers fail for other reasons. The only moral reason for drawing a distinction between the causes of liver failure is whether a particular disease state lessens treatment efficacy (Caplan, 1992a).

Still, as is true in many other areas of medicine, judgments about the virtue and vice of patients sometimes do enter into decisions about who will and will not receive care. As increasing emphasis is placed on the need to contain costs and decrease expenditures for health care, the role that personal responsibility plays in this equation will come in for greater scrutiny. If "sin" is not to become a standard applied at the bedside when decisions are made about who will live and who will die, then we must keep in mind how prevalent sin really is.

fourteen

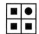

The Ethics of Gatekeepers

Cost Containment—A New Source of Moral Concern

HEALTH POLICY HAS TAKEN A SHARP TURN toward cost containment in the past few years. Efforts to use managed care, capitation, efficacy assessments, group purchasing, case management, utilization review, and restricted formularies to contain costs have been implemented in all parts of the country with great intensity. Attempts to implement federal and state solutions for regulating health care costs have sputtered. The solution seized upon by both the private and public sectors is the use of the private free market, often driven by the motive of profit, to constrain costs.

The sole goal of health care policy in the United States, at both the national and the state levels, is now the attainment of lower costs. The drive to use market strategies to solve the problem of cost has had a direct impact on the kinds of moral problems that face both providers and patients.

Americans are accustomed to worrying about whether doctors, chronic care facilities, hospitals, and pharmacists are perhaps doing too much to them in order to maximize their reimbursements. For decades for-fee medicine brought in its wake the worry that the doctor was doing too much—holding the patient another day in the hospital, ordering one more test, asking for one more evaluation—because it was in the provider's best fiscal interest to do more. The sicker someone was, the more desperate the situation, the more lucrative it was to provide care. The suspicion that more rather than less was being done was troubling, but in a culture that prefers more to less of almost everything and that sees doing more as doing better when it comes to health care, this was a problem that Americans could accept. Times have changed.

There is a real push in health care, most obviously manifest in the explosion of managed care, to control costs by doing less. There is now an attempt to make sure that each test is really needed, that people do not linger too long in the delivery room, intensive care unit, or recovery room, and that the cheapest effective drug or medical device is the one that is selected. Dying is no longer the source of revenue it once was, and all of a sudden more and more of us are going to hospice or our homes to die.

Americans are not at all accustomed to the idea of their doctor, hospital, or pharmacist doing less rather than more. The shift toward restraint is especially morally worrisome because it comes at a time when fewer and fewer Americans are permitted to have longstanding relationships with health care providers whom they know and trust. Managed care sometimes means a lack of continuity in care. Acute care almost always means a lack of continuity in care. Most of the fear in evidence about the morality of managed care swirls around the concern that not enough will be done in a system that rewards providers who are strangers for not being aggressive in diagnosis and treatment.

Providers feel the heat created by the shift in social priorities to containing costs. It is becoming increasingly obvious that the crucial moral challenge to those providing health care for the rest of this century and well into the next is how best to preserve professional integrity while trying to achieve greater efficiencies in the delivery of services in order to contain costs (Caplan, 1995b). If advocacy is crucial to the ethics of being a health care provider, then squaring advocacy with fiscal limits is the central moral challenge posed by the economic and institutional revolution in U.S. health care.

There is much dispute about the moral foundations that ought to underlie any attempt to contain costs. Recent writings have focused on various principles that ought to be invoked to guide hard choices about how to ration care. But battles over which rules or criteria should guide rationing are not the main moral dilemma raised by current efforts to contain costs.

Americans are notably unwilling, as are the citizens of most nations, to openly and publicly address the question of rationing. In fact, they may be more willing than most, since there was a brief and courageous experiment in community dialogue about rationing in the State of Oregon in the early part of this decade. But it spawned no imitators. The solution to ethical cost containment does not hinge upon the discovery of a set of public rules that all agree constitute fair recipes for rationing. No such rules are likely to command consensus, and they are even less likely to be adopted through the political process.

Approaches to rationing adopted in the United States are almost certain to leave decisions about constraining resources to those who deliver care at the bedside. The providers are expected to justify their decisions to their health care systems and provider organizations. The tension between the drive to force health care professionals to contain costs without compromising their professional responsibility to act as zealous advocates for commanding resources for those dependent on them for care is omnipresent within contemporary health care. It is the direct result of the desire to ration services without invoking an explicit public standard, without holding anyone to account for the choices that are made.

Using health care providers as gatekeepers comes at a high price. When rationing takes place at the bedside, moral questions erupt about the role of gatekeeper. Since large segments of the current system are run with an eye toward bottom-line concerns and the desire of stockholders to see earnings maximized, there is increasing concern about the compatibility of business ethics with health care ethics when those at the bedside are forced to make hard choices about the allocation of resources.

Ethics in an Age of Cost Containment

Health care has always faced issues of resource constraint and limits. For most patients it is always the case that a little bit more might be done. Another week or two or ten of physical therapy might help the stroke patient regain just a little bit more function. One more x-ray or lab test might reveal something of importance. Another day in the NICU might do the preemie baby some good. Since a tiny bit more could always in theory be done, there never seem to be sufficient beds or providers to care for those who have suffered disabling diseases and disorders.

Managed care is not the source of the role of money in steering the kinds of choices that are made in medicine and health care. Money has always played a role in health care.

Issues of when to initiate care and when to stop it have hinged in part on issues of insurance coverage and the ability of patients to pay for care. Those who can pay have historically had better access to services. The ability to pay has long driven decisions about who should be admitted to hospitals, chronic and long-term care, how long they stay there, what happens when they are there and where they go next upon discharge.

But the forces that drove the economics of health care are changing. Today providers complain that patients are being discharged too quickly because this is often a cheaper alternative for a third-party payer than having patients remain in acute care settings. Families of patients requiring chronic care increasingly find themselves challenged to provide more kinds of care by themselves in their homes. "Sicker but quicker" is a phrase that is often heard in health care settings these days.

Advocacy Endangered

Physicians and nurses are taught early in their medical careers that their primary moral responsibility is to the patient. Zealous advocacy is an expected virtue on the part of every physician in terms of securing resources for those in their care (Spece, Shimm, and Buchanan, 1996). Doctors and nurses must act in their patient's best interest as the patient defines that interest. Abandonment of the patient is the worst moral sin a health care provider can commit.

When society decides that costs must be constrained and institutes methods of financing or health care delivery aimed at achieving these goals, public policy has often turned to the physician as the person who must control access to resources in the name of the hospital, corporation, health plan, payer, or society. The same physician is often left morally ambivalent and conflicted about guarding the gate to protect economic resources while at the same time feeling a professional duty to advocate for the needs of patients who seek to use those resources for their own needs. When society asks health care providers to think about discharging patients who might be able to make more progress because an insurance plan will pay for only so many days of care, these are constraints that are hard to square, morally, with the duty to be a zealous patient advocate (Baer, Fagin, and Gordon, 1996).

Health care is a field that has recently begun to celebrate the fact that its services are delivered by teams rather than by any single provider or specialty. But in an era of cost containment, teams sometimes appear to be unaffordable luxuries. Professional integrity about how best to provide services is constantly under challenge in environments in which every team member is constantly challenged to prove his or her value, not only in terms of outcome but in terms of dollars, in the care of every single patient.

Patients and their families are also facing new moral dilemmas as fiscal constraints impact team-oriented health care. When the fiscal goal is to keep expenditures in check and the means to do so involves different forms of managed care and physician gatekeeping, then families begin to wonder who on the team is really in charge and who in particular on the team is looking out for their interests. It is harder to know who is at the gate when a team is providing care (Baer and Gordon, 1994).

A crucial element in any therapeutic relationship is trust. Physician advocacy is important not just to command the requisite resources for patients who cannot do so on their own but also to cement trust between doctor and patient. Trust is the basis for the honest and frank exchange of information and for the patient's willingness to believe that healing and recovery will result from the physicians' and therapists' ministrations. Trust is weakened or evaporates because patients are no longer sure whether the person minding the gate of health care resources is looking out for their interests or is more concerned about the interests, fiscal and otherwise, of third parties.

Does a Free-Market Approach Square with Virtue?

Markets oriented to the bottom line do some things well. They can provide resources efficiently in response to consumer demand. However, they fail dismally at achieving other ends. The promulgation of virtue is one area where markets may fail. Recent events in the world of professional sports provide a useful lesson in what markets can do to imperil virtue.

The Browns, a professional football team, played for decades in Cleveland. But the team is now playing in Baltimore under the name of the Ravens. Many people in Cleveland were distraught about the move by the Browns. They felt their team was disloyal. How could the Browns ignore decades of tradition and fan support and simply jump at a more lucrative offer? Some Browns fans, like some fans of the Baltimore Colts, a team that snuck away from Baltimore in the middle of the night when the team's owner received an attractive bid to move from a group of investors in Indianapolis, say that they cannot put their trust in professional sports franchises that pick up and move whenever a better deal appears on the horizon. The same distrust is in evidence in baseball, where many fans, embittered by a prolonged strike and seemingly endless labor negotiations, are staying away from ball parks in significant numbers.

Some respond that football and baseball at the professional level are businesses. But those who follow professional football, baseball, or basketball do not follow them because they are businesses. They follow them for very different reasons, primarily for what they offer in the way of virtue. Sports is an arena of life where hard work, fidelity, loyalty, dogged-ness, accountability, and enthusiasm count, or at least those who are fans want them to count. Money is corrosive to the belief in these virtues. When money is revealed to be the only force driving the behavior of those involved in professional sports, fans begin to lose interest.

What does this have to do with health care ethics? Plenty. Why are sports fans upset about the relocations in football or labor battles in baseball or the movement of key players from one town to another in basketball and other professional sports? They are angry owing to market failure. In professional sports the market is now saying that if you have a team or a star and someone else has more money, "your" team or star will move if the price is right. There is no such thing as loyalty, fidelity, a sense of community. In short, when the market drives behavior it is very difficult for trust to survive.

Virtues do not thrive in bottom-line, profit-oriented markets. The market in professional sports is distributing teams efficiently, but it is not giving fans what they want: teams to which they can feel loyal and have that loyalty reciprocated. If a bottom-line orientation does not support virtue in sports, is there any reason to presume it will preserve the virtues people even more fervently expect and need from their health care providers and institutions?

Many of the features that providers and patients want from their medical providers and facilities are not likely to be present in a purely economically oriented free-market system. Big corporations that lack local ties are more attentive to the fiscal concerns of their investors than they are to the specific local concerns of any facility or family. Just as is true with sports teams, CEOs and hospital management companies can move facilities, close them, or downsize them as the bottom line dictates. Administrators can order doctors and nurses and therapists to change the way they practice, with attention only on the economic consequences of practice, not the moral compromise such emphases sometimes entail for the provider. They can make it clear that criticism of the organization, especially with patients, will come with a significant price tag, as efforts to impose gag rules in many managed care organizations make clear. It is hard to trust or exhibit loyalty toward a large corporation whose chief officers make hundreds of millions of dollars and whose contact with providers and patients is limited to reviews of ledger sheets.

An unregulated market confronts patients with a system whose savings are great but whose virtues are few. If the patients being cared for are especially disabled, frail, and vulnerable, then the absence of virtue will prove especially bothersome to both providers and patients in these settings. For patients, putting trust in advocates whose virtues are suspect because their conduct seems driven by attention to the bottom line will be a difficult thing to do (Spece, Shimm, and Buchanan, 1996).

Who Is That at the Gate?

The shift to cost constraint as the main goal of health policy and the demand that providers conserve or skimp on resources exemplified by some forms of managed care, case management, and other capitated forms of health care reimbursement lead to a different but still troubling dilemma for the provider at the gate charged with being both a good advocate and a responsible steward of the resources on the other side of the gate. How far ought a doctor or nurse or social worker go to stretch the truth in the name of swinging open the gate?

If a patient needs a special piece of equipment or another day on the floor prior to discharge, does the virtuous health care provider upgrade a diagnosis, fudge a test result, color a DRG category in a different way, or lie about a prognosis? An example of how access to specific benefits hinges on the willingness of health care providers to compromise some values in the name of advocacy may show how important it is that in a world in which cost containment is king, a bit of subversion may be required if patients' needs are to be met.

A few years ago, when a person who was enrolled in a large HMO was receiving care in a long-term care setting and wanted to use an experimental procedure to relieve pain, I had the chance to sit in on a meeting where the request for approval to pay for this experimental procedure was considered. The medical director explained to the board of directors of the health plan that Mr. Smith needed a new and complicated form of treatment. The director went on to note that Smith's physicians believed the procedure was necessary and therapeutic. He then observed that the procedure had never been tried before in this state and that as far as he knew only three exactly like it in similar patients had been done in the United States. He felt that there was no reason to expect the new procedure would work but that the board had to take the request seriously because of the positive opinions offered by Smith's doctors.

The first question from the board of directors was "Does Mr. Smith have a lawyer?" The second was "Is Mr. Smith articulate?" The third question was "Is Mr. Smith likely to cause a problem if we turn him down—will he appear on television?" No one questioned the assertion of the doctors that a new procedure would work or was even properly thought of as therapeutic. The answers to the questions were all "yes" and Mr. Smith got coverage for his treatment.

This is not a fair way to allocate scare resources. In fact, it is a morally repugnant approach. Combinations of threats and wheel-squeaking behavior place those who know how or are willing to do these things at a great advantage in capturing scarce resources. Those who are shy, lack family and friends, are kids, are disabled, or are simply inarticulate lose.

The case also shows that battles at the gate over what is available in terms of coverage also obligate health care providers to sometimes say things they know not to be exactly true in the name of advocacy. Any system or mode of allocation that requires systematic dishonesty in the name of advocacy as a constant feature of professionalism is a system at severe risk, compromising the integrity of its professionals. Dissembling, even if required by patient interests, does not sit comfortably with virtue for long.

Is a Bottom-Line Orientation Ethical?

Patients who receive their care in for-profit managed care systems are at a severe disadvantage. They must surrender their privacy in the interests of efficiency as managers insist on seeing every detail concerning their care. Informed consent is compromised, since in tightly managed systems of health care, patients must waive all rights to privacy and confidentiality as a condition of receiving coverage.

Patients may not know that the providers giving them care have their own conflicts of interest about when to continue care and when to stop it. If providers are prohibited from speaking openly and honestly, presenting all therapeutic options, directing patients to providers or facilities outside the plan, explaining their financial incentives and payment arrangements, or even criticizing what is in the formulary or the competencies of agencies used to provide various services, then informed consent is meaningless. So too is any notion of consumer choice.

In much of managed care in many parts of the United States, many must use the systems that they are given by the government or their employers. Choice of provider is for large numbers of Americans an illusion. Most people have no choice but to go with the coverage that their employer provides. If they or a dependent suddenly need specialized services, they may not be able to change jobs or health plans.

Restrictions on choice in the real world are not confined to provider or plan. Patients often must live with the doctor, nurse, or team that is assigned to them. If a particular doctor leaves a plan or a network, then the ability to see that provider is severely restricted. In such circumstances, the goals of treatment may be set by people whom the patient and family do not know, who lack a longstanding relationship with the patient, and whom they cannot call readily to account for crucial decisions about their medical treatment.

Under profit-driven managed care, the incentives have shifted. Now efficiency and profit margins loom in the calculus of what services are provided and who provides them. Relatively little data is available to patients or even to providers. But financial incentives do influence what doctors and nurses do. The only way to protect patient interests is to insist that virtues and professional integrity not be sacrificed in the name of cost. If gatekeeping is to become a part of the ethos of health care in the United States, then it ought not come to the bedside.

Preserving Professional Integrity

It will not do for those in health care to rent their garments and loudly lament the loss of autonomy and control that some new efforts at cost containment represent. The American people want costs constrained. But they do not want to lose trust in their doctors, nurses, social workers, physical and occupational therapists. Those in health care must make the case that cost containment efforts, be they for-profit managed care or other strategies, that compromise their ability to advocate zealously for those in their care are immoral and unacceptable. They must make this case to administrators, the public, and legislators. Decisions about benefits and coverage must be made in an open and accountable manner. Limits should rarely be set at the bedside by clinical providers. They ought be set far from the clinical setting by boards and panels that have input from patients and their families as well as providers.

Those who receive care should have some say over what is provided to them. Those who set limits on what is available should be accountable to more than their stockholders when the service they are marketing is health care. Decisions about limits and coverage boundaries should be made in public forums where decisions can be scrutinized and those who make them held to account.

Further, there should be a political mechanism in place to make sure that every coverage decision and resource determination is accountable. Accountability is especially crucial when the recipients of health care are disabled, severely impaired, or institutionalized.

There is nothing intrinsically wrong with trying to make money out of health care. But decisions about major resource constraints must be made by someone besides the provider of care. It is immoral to place the burden of gatekeeping solely on the provider at the bedside, because to do so places in jeopardy the very virtues essential for the successful practice of health care. Healing requires trust. Health care ethics must place the virtues requisite for trust at the core of the duties owed to those who require care. In the short run it is easier for society to ask those at the bedside to make the hard choices about how to ration services. In the long run, if those at the bedside are the only persons responsible for making these decisions, the bedside will be seen as a frightening place to be by both providers and patients.

PART FIVE

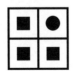

WHAT IS YOUR
DOCTOR TRYING TO
DO TO YOU?

fifteen

Who Says You're Sick?

ENORMOUS SUMS OF MONEY—IN THE UNITED STATES more than a trillion dollars in 1996—are spent on health care. The nations of Western Europe, Scandinavia, Canada, Australia, New Zealand, Korea, Singapore, and Japan spend thousands of dollars per person annually for medical care and other health-related activities. Many persons devote large amounts of their time to the pursuit of behaviors and lifestyles which they believe will enhance their health and stave off disease.

The analysis of the concepts of health, illness, and disease is not a mere exercise in intellectual inquiry. Decisions about the meaning of these terms have direct and important consequences for daily life and the allocation of vast amounts of social resources.

The concepts of health and disease, as well as the persons and institutions concerned with them, did not always play such central roles in human affairs. As recently as the mid–nineteenth century, physicians and hospitals occupied minor, peripheral roles. Few persons actively pursued health by means of lifestyle, diet, or daily regimens of any sort. It is not clear that they could. The prevailing notions of health and wellness, what they meant and why they existed, were not especially amenable to conscious pursuit by individuals. Health was more often seen as a reflection of divine favor or simple luck than anything else.

Prior to this century, disease was feared and stigmatized; it was rarely the object of ministration by organized medicine or health care institutions. Laymen, family, and clerics were where the sick turned. The situation today has changed radically. Why is this so, and why do these concepts play such a central role in contemporary life?

The emergent concern with health and disease in this century is a function of many forces. The conquest of the pain associated with medical treatment, especially surgery, in the late nineteenth century by means of anesthesia and anesthetics played a key role. The demonstrable efficacy of twentieth-century medicine and public health in preventing or reversing many forms of infection, dysfunction, and nutritional deficiency are important reasons for the prominence of concerns about health and disease. Modern ways of conceiving disease, such as germ theory, the role of toxic exposure in damaging health, and the genetic basis of many diseases, compelled changes in the understanding of what disease and health mean from the viewpoint of prophylaxis and cure. It was not, however, simply the success enjoyed by medicine and its attendant conceptual models of health and disease over the past one hundred years that brought the concepts of health and disease center stage.

The historic connection in many theological writings, particularly Protestant ones, between health and moral character has played a key role in establishing the cultural importance of health and disease in Western societies. Disease and disability have been seen by many religious traditions as reflections of God's displeasure with sin and with the impure in mind if not in actual deed. The current interest in health and the prevention and avoidance of disease reflects the legacy of conceiving of disease and illness as instruments of divine displeasure. Many believe that if they are sick somehow they are responsible, and if they fail to get well it is because they did not do enough to earn a reprieve from God, the saints, or various other supernatural entities (Sigerist, 1943; Szusz, 1961).

In a Western world grown far more secular in this century, at least in its public culture, disease, disability, and health have become transformed. Disease is no longer a sign of divine displeasure or a mark of sin. Disease is not seen as having instrumental value; it has intrinsic importance. Health, in itself, is a sign of good moral character and individual worth, whereas disease is equated with moral failure. Those who are fat or who smoke are not merely imprudent—they are bad. Those who die of AIDS or cancer did not think positively enough or pray hard enough.

As the prospects for the control of illness and disease increased, the causal locus of the origins of disease began to shift toward the individual rather than outside forces or agents. This shift brought in its wake a shift toward the equation of health with good character and virtuous conduct When those with cancer are told to use their mental powers to visualize malignant cells in order to slow their spread, when female workers are told they cannot hold jobs in a particular factory because the chemicals present pose risks to their motherhood, when individuals are told they can use laughter or will power to reverse the course of disease, when experts and celebrities demand the control of diet, exercise, stress, or sexuality as the key to good health, then disease and health have taken a highly individualistic focus and thus are direct means for assessing the moral worth and value of human beings. Secularized medicine and its theories have taken on the role once played by religion in explaining disease and health.

Technology also has had a role in the emergence of health and disease as central cultural concerns in the Western world. As nineteenth-century science, especially under the influence of Darwinism, began to diminish the boundaries that had made human beings seem special and unique among living things, medicine became more willing to treat human beings as possible objects for scientific scrutiny and technologically based intervention.

Throughout the twentieth century and particularly after the Second World War, technology came to play an increasingly important role in our health care system. This is reflected in the emphasis in many modern health care delivery systems on the treatment of acute medical problems in hospital settings. The proliferation of neonatal units, CAT and PET scanners, ultrasound, laser surgery, adult ICUs, and organ and tissue transplants is a reflection of our collective faith in the power of technology and our belief that it can be used to identify and control the evils of disease and disability. Technology has reified health and disease; it has made it seem as if diseases are real entities in the world that can be observed, identified, manipulated, controlled, and eliminated (Foucault, 1965).

Prior to the First World War, there was relatively little that physicians or anyone else could do to combat the effects of acute disease and severe disability. The introduction of antibiotics, vaccines, transfusions, powerful diagnostic technologies and technologically based therapies in the decades following the war transformed medicine from a profession focused on diagnosis and caring to one with a serious interest in curing. The expectations of physicians and patients have grown considerably and, as a result, the desire to be returned to a state of health after the onset of disease or injury seems as much a matter of finding a competent professional or getting into the latest research study as it is a matter for hope, wishes, and prayers.

Nowhere is so much attention devoted to health as in the United States. Particular political, economic, and social values place a special premium on health and the avoidance of disease in this society.

Health and the alleviation of disease and disability have key roles to play in highly competitive, capitalist societies. Societies committed to free-market economics can tolerate significant differences in the resources and statuses held by individual citizens. Such differences can only be accepted, however, if there is a general acceptance of the means by which resources were acquired and held. A concern for equality of opportunity in economic life in many countries leads inevitably to the assignment of great weight to the preservation of health and the prevention of disease and disability.

The moral assessment of inequalities of power, possessions, and property is contingent upon the view that prevails of the opportunities that have preceded the creation of inequities in the distribution of social goods. If some people are rich because they work hard and others are poor because they are lazy, then so be it. As long as a relative equality of opportunity exists, as long as the initial conditions for competing economically are seen as fair, then any differences that result are easier to accept on moral grounds.

If equality of opportunity is a critical moral component of the legal, political, and societal norms of free-market societies, then health and disease will be accorded special status. Those who are born with congenital deformities and those who suffer from disabling or chronic diseases, especially if they are infants or children, cannot be said to have an equal opportunity to compete with their peers for the goods and benefits that a competitive society makes available. The alleviation of disease and disability and the promotion of health are important political and cultural goals for the same reasons special priority is given to the provision of basic education, shelter, and food. All of these factors influence the extent to which equality can legitimately be said to exist with respect to opportunities and therefore to the extent to which the inequalities that result from a free-market approach to the distribution of social resources can be viewed as morally palatable.

Disease and disability become the object of concern in Western society, especially in the United States, because they are seen as threats to equal opportunity and, in turn, to the moral foundation of economic life. Unless the moral suppositions of U.S. society are part of the equation, the dominance of medicine as a source of power and authority cannot be explained. The reductions in abilities and capacities that usually accompany diseases are threatening not only because they cause intrinsic harms to those beset by them but also because they undermine the social commitment to the equity of competition and the fairness of the market as efficient methods for distributing social resources. Even though it may be expensive to redress the effects of disease or to prevent its occurrence, if fundamental inequities exist among people because of serious but remediable differences in their health and well-being, this is a state of affairs that is incompatible with a socioeconomic orientation that seeks to reward striving, performance, and individual achievement. Economics plays a major role in thrusting the concepts of health and disease center stage in developed nations that are organized around competitive markets.

Health, Disease, and the Scope of Medicine

If it is true that health and disease play powerful roles in filling important gaps left by the secularization of public culture and in legitimizing key presuppositions of prevailing socioeconomic arrangements in the United States, it is obvious why so much attention has centered in recent decades on their meaning and definition. The definitions accorded these concepts play pivotal roles in establishing the boundaries of access to the health care system, the limits of medical concern and professional control, and the extent of the obligation to share in the burden of alleviating disease, disability, and dysfunction.

Prima facie obligations exist for government to correct the inequalities wrought by disease and illness. Thus the definition of these terms is more than a philosophical exercise. The answer to the question of what does or does not constitute a disease will determine not only how much authority or power is available to those responsible for alleviating the consequences of disease—physicians, nurses, public health officials, social workers, and other health care professionals—but what government must do to shift resources toward those with special needs resulting from ill health in order to make economic and social life fair.

There has been much concern on the part of a variety of social commentators and ethicists from both ends of the political spectrum about the growing power and influence of medicine and other health care professions in our society. Conservatives worry, for example, that physicians, nurses, and psychologists will introduce adolescent students to permissive attitudes toward sexual conduct in the guise of promoting health education. Liberals fear, for instance, that the classification of homosexuality as a disease rather than a matter of biological necessity will result in discriminatory treatment of homosexuals and the promotion of negative stereotypes. The definitions of health, disease, and illness are seen by many as political issues, requiring input from both professionals and lay persons (Baxter, 1981; Caplan, Engelhardt, McCartney, 1981).

Physicians are now able to control access to a wide variety of social and economic resources by the use of their authority as gatekeepers of eligibility for a wide spectrum of public and private programs. Getting a job, receiving life insurance, permission to immigrate, admission to school, entry into and out of the armed services, access to legal compensation, exculpation from crime, the ability to marry and to have and raise a family are all controlled to some extent by physicians and other health care professionals. Similarly, decisions about who will or will not be forced to receive medical care in hospital or institutional settings, who is or is not free to refuse medication or confinement, and what is or is not an acceptable form of medical treatment are controlled by physicians and other health care personnel (Foucault, 1965).

Physicians and other health care providers not only have the authority to enfranchise some members of society with social benefits or privileges; they also have the authority to excuse behavior that, without medical exculpation, might be the object of police, judicial, or penal attention. Many groups have fought long and hard to have particular behavioral dispositions labeled as diseases. Alcoholics, gamblers, and those with chronic back pain are but a few of the groups who have lobbied persistently to have their conditions labeled as diseases. The disease label excuses certain behavior that might otherwise he viewed as criminal, sinful, or lazy and thus be subject to various forms of sanction.

Conversely, many groups, such as homosexuals and the disabled, have struggled to free themselves from being categorized as ill or diseased. Disease labels, while often exculpatory in terms of liability or responsibility, carry other burdens, such as the stigma attached to illness and the assumption that those who are ill or diseased require treatment and cure from legitimate experts (Baxter, 1981; Pellegrino and Thomasma, 1988).

If the scope and domain of medicine and the related healing arts are to be accurately delineated, a clear understanding of the concepts of health and disease is a necessity. The definitions that are given to these concepts are critical both for understanding the possibilities and limits of health care and for understanding the moral obligations, rights, and responsibilities that ought to prevail between patients and providers in health care contexts.

The Relationship between the Concepts of Health and Disease

What is the nature of the logical relationship between health, illness, and disease? Many health care professionals and a large percentage of the general public appear to view health and disease as logical opposites, while illness and disease are often used as synonyms. When asked if they are healthy or feel well, most people will answer affirmatively if they are not suffering from any particular disease or disorder at the time the question is asked. Looked at uncritically, health would seem to be no more than the absence of disease and illness. Disease and illness appear to connote any impairment in a person's sense of well-being or fitness.

But there are powerful reasons for questioning the appropriateness of viewing health and disease merely as conceptual opposites and disease and illness as synonyms. Even if no particular disease is present, it is still possible to say that a person seems healthier or is healthier in certain ways than others. The average marathon runner or professional athlete is, with respect to overall physical well-being, probably healthier than the average philosophy professor, even if neither happens to be afflicted with a specific disease at the time the comparison is made.

Health does seem to require the absence of disease or illness as a necessary condition. But it is not clear that this absence is by itself sufficient to define the nature of health.

The possibility that health is not simply the absence of disease or illness but refers to something more is reinforced by the activities of some contemporary health care practitioners. Some see their job as more than simply the alleviation of disease. Psychoanalysts, plastic surgeons, nutritionists, and sports physiologists are interested not only in the prevention or alleviation of disease but also, and perhaps sometimes only, in the promotion of health. If health and disease were logically related to one another as contradictory concepts, it would be impossible to make any sense of the ideas expressed by such terms as *maximizing health* and *positive mental health*. These ideas, as well as the notion that relative degrees of health can exist even in the absence of disease or illness, do appear to be meaningful and coherent.

Not only is the absence of disease not sufficient to establish the existence of health; diseases do not always impair or threaten health. Some diseases are unpleasant and disabling but do not compromise the health of the individual who has them. For example, enduring a short bout of the measles or mumps during childhood, either through infection or inoculation, may actually be conducive to health. A person can be riddled with cancer, be delusional, or suffer from hypertension and yet remain entirely unaware of any symptoms or dysfunction. A person who is the carrier of the sickle cell trait, while prone to certain problems under certain rare circumstances, is better protected against malaria than someone lacking this genetic endowment.

The fact that one can be functioning well and feel healthy while suffering from a disease also hints that the concepts of illness and disease may actually refer to different states or conditions. Feeling sick is not the same as having a disease, since one can be ill but not diseased and diseased but not feel ill (Murphy, 1976; Caplan, Engelhardt, McCartney, 1981).

Some behaviors that are viewed as diseases in some circles—gambling, homosexuality, hyperactivity, drug addiction—have tenuous logical connections to the concept of health. Certainly it is much less difficult to obtain agreement across social classes and different cultures about those states of the mind and body that constitute diseases than it is to secure agreement about which states are to be viewed as healthy. The use of addictive narcotic drugs and its relationship to health is viewed quite differently in Jamaica, Holland, Bolivia, and Peru than it is in the United States and Saudi Arabia.

While the view of health and disease as conceptual opposites may be widely accepted, there are reasons for calling this presumption into question. A strong case can be made for the view that the logical relationship between health and disease is not one of contradiction. The conceptual opposite of health might more reasonably be seen as unhealthy and the logical contradictory of diseased as nondiseased. Health and disease may exist as parallel concepts rather than as concepts defined only in terms of one another. While disease may be among the criteria that are used to define health, other measures or states may be necessary in order to attribute this state to an individual and vice versa (Resnek, 1987).

Normativism versus Nonnormativism in the Definition of Disease

Perhaps the major point of contention among philosophers, physicians, and other health care experts who have examined the meaning of health and disease is the extent to which value judgments are requisite for or are implicit in the definitions of these concepts. Many physicians and not a few philosophers believe that there is no need to resort to considerations of value in general or morality in particular to identify, understand, or analyze the concepts of health, illness, and disease. Those who subscribe to nonnormativism believe that determinations of health and disease are matters of empirical fact and nothing more.

One way in which the case for assigning a key role to values in the definition of health and disease is made by those who espouse the contrary view, normativism—to observe that categories of disease vary from culture to culture and historical period to historical period. Moreover, what is supposed to be the same disease or the same state of health can produce very different experiences in different people.

Granted, not everyone has the same experience in conjunction with disease. One common way of responding to this fact is to use the term *illness* to refer to the subjective perception or the phenomenological experience of disease. If anxiety causes some individuals to hyperventilate but causes a tightening sensation in the chest of others and a headache in still other persons, this wide range of symptoms, responses, and experiences can be captured by the term *illness*.

Illness is by definition subjective and thus specific to time, place, and culture. Variations in illness are to be expected. It seems beyond dispute that illness, defined only as the experience of health or disease, is heavily influenced by the prevailing values and norms of a given society. Indeed, those who wish to defend the view that health and disease can be defined in purely objective terms without reference to values are more than willing to concede the historical and sociological findings of Foucault, Gilman, Szasz, Sedgwick, and Canguilhem that disease is irremediably a product of culture, economics, and ideology. However, by segregating the perception of disease and the response a disease elicits in a particular individual living in a particular society under the rubric of illness, those who seek a nonnormative definition hope to be able to find univocal meanings for disease (and sometimes for health) that transcend the specifics of time, place, and person.

What is at stake in the battle over the role played by values is the objectivity of claims about disease and health. If values play crucial roles in shaping the meanings of not only illness but also health and disease, then it appears as if the prospects for objectivity in medicine and health care, which depend upon these concepts, are imperiled. If values infuse the analysis of disease, then diseases seem to be a product of human invention. Diseases would be categories imposed by human beings upon human beings, not states which they possess and which can be discovered by anyone who has learned the criteria and evidence requisite to making a diagnosis. The greater the role of values in the definition of health and disease, the worse the prognosis appears to be for both their objectivity and reality. Ideology and politics loom especially large in the classification of human behaviors and states as indicative of health or disease as soon as values appear, since values, unlike empirical facts, are seen very much as products of social forces. And if disease and health are matters of ideology and politics, then the prospects for an objective, verifiable science of medicine seem diminished, if not simply hopeless.

The clearest contemporary expression of the view that health and disease can be defined without explicit reference to moral values or ethical norms has been offered by the American philosopher Christopher Boorse (Boorse, 1975, 1976, 1987). He argues that while it is true that different social, ethnic, and economic groups do not agree on the reference class of the terms *health* and *disease,* and while it is also true that professionals often disagree about the disease status of a particular condition or behavior, it would be wrong to conclude from such facts that an objective definition of health or disease that does not rely on values is impossible to attain.

Boorse contends that while different people or groups do disagree about the specific application of a disease definition to particular cases, this does nothing to disprove the possibility of locating an objective, value-free definition of disease. Illness is often subjective and variable. Disease need not be.

All organisms, including human beings, are the product of a long course of biological evolution. Human evolution has been driven by a wide variety of environmental demands that have conferred advantages on those creatures possessing certain phenotypic and genotypic traits. Since our minds and bodies have evolved in response to our evolutionary past, health consists in our functioning in conformity with our natural design as determined by natural selection.

If kidneys exist as a result of evolving in response to the contingent forces of natural selection so that their function is to remove impurities from the body, if hearts evolved to pump blood to organs and tissues, if external ears evolved in order to allow the localization of sound, then in any human being (or any other organism for that matter) possessing kidneys, heart, or ears, health consists, in part, in having a kidney that removes impurities from the blood, a heart that pumps blood to organs and tissues, and ears that can localize sounds. These organs were designed by evolution to perform such functions, and when they do so, the organism that possesses them can be said to be healthy. If they do them especially well, regardless of why that is so, the person who owns them can be said to have a very healthy heart or an especially sound pair of kidneys.

If there is some failure in an organ system, if it loses the capacity to perform the function for which it was designed by evolution to perform, this is indicative of disease, whether it is perceived as illness or not. Natural design permits an analysis of health or disease independent of the experience of the person. Illness but not disease is in the mind of the beholder. Values need not enter into the definition of the concepts of health and disease at all. This is because the goals that drive evolution have nothing to do with ethics, morals, ideology, sociology, or values.

Evolution places a premium on survival and reproduction. Survival and reproduction are the only goals that matter for evolution. In order to attain these goals, all organisms, including humans, have evolved traits that increase the probability of their survival and the transmission of their genes into the next generation. Organisms that lacked the genotypes and phenotypes requisite for survival and reproduction are extinct. Only those with traits adequate for survival and reproduction are here today.

Disease can be defined as any impairment of the functions typical of a particular biological species, functions required to achieve the natural goals set not by politics or culture but by the twin demands of survival and reproduction. Are concepts such as survival and reproduction themselves value laden? Neither of these concepts is used in any moralistic or evaluative sense—survival and reproduction are merely the contingent by-products of a Darwinian system responding to a specific set of historical circumstances. There is nothing good or bad about them—they merely exist.

If one accepts the view that the goals of survival and reproduction have guided the evolution of every living organism on this planet, then health and disease can be understood solely in terms of the causal contributions various states, conditions, and behaviors make to the achievement of these ends. No resort to ethics or any other sort of value judgment is necessary. All that must be done is to determine whether the causal contribution of a particular trait or behavior is positive or negative in terms of the overall capacity of a particular organism to achieve its biologically designed ends. The extent to which this is so determines whether or not the trait or behavior is to be classified as healthy or diseased.

An especially persuasive argument that values need play no role in the definitions of health and disease is that a nonnormative analysis works as well for assessing the health status of plants and animals as it does for humans. Veterinarians know what it means for a cat or a pig to be sick. Few would want to argue that before they could say that an animal was sick or dying, they must resort to an examination of the animal's mores or understand the animal's values!

Health as Normality, Disease as Abnormality

Non-normativism, the position that disease can be defined without reference to anything other than the empirical assessment of functions based solely upon the understanding of the purposes that the functions were designed to serve, is closely related to the definitions of health and disease used in contemporary medical texts. Many physicians, if pressed to define health and disease, will respond that disease is anything that is abnormal and health is what is normal.

Normal and abnormal refer to statistical normalcy, not any sort of value judgment about a particular state or behavior. The unusual, the uncommon, and the extreme become candidates for classification as disease. Those states and behaviors that cluster around the mean or for which there is relatively small variance become the reference class of health.

The statistical conception of health and disease has prevailed in Western medicine for many decades. It is a legacy of the ancient theory of humors and the more modern conception of balance, or homeostasis, which grounded thinking about health and disease for many centuries. Health for thinkers as diverse as Galen of Pergamum, William Cullen, and Walter B. Cannon consisted in the attainment of a balance or harmony in the workings of the body. Deviations or abnormalities in the composition of bodily fluids or, in later times, organ systems connoted disease (Scadding, 1967, 1996).

Physicians often do equate abnormal measures of blood pressure, blood chemistry, or body weight with disease—regardless of whether dysfunction or pain are present. The primary problem with the attempt to establish a value-free definition of both health and disease is that anything "unusual" is considered a disease state, even when it is not at all clear why it is unhealthy to be abnormal. It seems conceptually bizarre to say that the unusually tall, intelligent, strong, fast, or agile are diseased simply by dint of their abnormality or deviance. Those at the tail ends of the distribution of any state, trait, or behavior would by definition be diseased, an analysis that seems too inclusive and at the same time indifferent to historical attempts to connect difference with dysfunction (Murphy, 1976).

The problem raised by the advantages conferred by some forms of statistical deviancy for the statistical approach to the definition of health and disease is serious. Abnormality is a sign or indication that something may be wrong, but it does not seem in and of itself to constitute disease. If a value-free conception of these concepts is to be found, it would seem that the attempt to root disease and health in a functional analysis, perhaps based upon the recognition that human beings are biological organisms that have evolved to meet the challenges of a shifting set of environmental demands, has the best chance of succeeding.

The Proponents of Normativism

Normativists believe that health and disease are concepts that are inherently value laden. They believe that to understand exactly what it is that these concepts mean or refer to, it is necessary to realize that decisions have to be made about states of the body or mind that must involve considerations of what is desirable or undesirable, useful or useless, good or bad. Normativists argue that no matter how many descriptive facts are known about the body or about the functions of a particular cell or organ system, it is impossible to decide whether or not a particular state of affairs represents health or disease without some reference to values (Szusz, 1961).

Historically, the primary focus of philosophical attention on the part of physicians and others interested in health care has been the concept of disease. If disease could be adequately defined and interpreted, then it was believed that all other questions about the aims, goals, and purposes of health care would be resolved.

Normativism is sometimes confused with alternative forms of healing. While there are some exponents of normativism in the ranks of those who espouse holistic health or alternative forms of medical intervention such as spiritual or psychic healing, most normativists are only concerned to defend the position that values form an irreducible element in the definition of disease.

Perhaps the clearest illustration of the ways in which values influence the definition of health and disease emerges from the realm of mental health and mental illness. A cursory glance at nineteenth-century American medical texts reveals that some physicians asserted with all of the authority at their disposal that women who enjoyed sexual intercourse or engaged in masturbation were afflicted with various forms of mental illness and often a variety of corresponding physical ailments as well. Textbooks of the era were replete with diseases of the mind that seemed to afflict only black men and women in astounding numbers. One omnipresent disorder of the day was a condition labeled drapetomania, a horrible plague that denoted an obsessive desire on the part of a slave to run away from his or her owner.

Normativists are much impressed with illustrations of the ways in which values and cultural prejudices tacitly or even overtly influence medical determinations of health and disease. They point to contemporary disputes about the disease status of such conditions as homosexuality, premenstrual syndrome, and infertility and ask how anyone could possibly conclude that labeling some particular physical or mental state as diseased or healthy involves nothing more than an empirical assessment of biological functioning (Bayer, 1981).

Both historical and contemporary cases of shifts in beliefs or uncertainties as to the proper classification of various conditions make it clear that values play an inextricable but entirely appropriate role in defining health and disease. Moreover, as normativists point out, a key element of the definition of disease is that the states of the body and mind that are viewed as diseases in various cultures are so viewed only as a result of the fact that people disvalue them.

In a society burdened with overpopulation, infertility might be viewed as a healthy state. In a society wealthy enough to provide financial support for all newborns and a bias toward large families, infertility might be seen as a disease state meriting serious attempts at amelioration through surgical or pharmacological intervention.

One of the boldest attempts to formulate a normative definition of disease highlights the valuational dimension of this concept. The psychiatrist Charles Culver and the philosopher Bernard Gert argue that the core meaning of disease involves the recognition that something is wrong with a person. They argue that diseases are actually a subcategory of a more general category which they label "maladies." The members of this class include not only diseases but also injuries, disabilities, and death itself. They argue that what is common to all these conditions is that human beings universally view them as evils. Other things being equal, people disvalue these states and try to avoid them if they can (Culver and Gert, 1982).

Unlike most nonnormative analyses of health and disease, which view disease and health in terms of deviations from statistical normalcy or from various norms of species typical functioning, Culver's and Gert's position is that it is not dysfunction but the perceived evil associated with dysfunction that is at the heart of understanding the meaning of disease. In the case of a myocardial infarct, it is not the deviation from normal functioning that makes us classify this event as a disease. Rather it is the loss of capacities, the onset of pain, and the risk to life itself, the evils associated with this dysfunction, that lead to the disvaluation of this particular deviation from functional normality.

While the members of different cultural groups or societies may not always agree on what constitutes an evil, every society recognizes certain states of the mind or body as evils to be avoided. While people may not always agree as to the identity of those mental or physical states that represent evils, most recognize that pain and death and the loss of abilities, freedom, or pleasure are evils. Malady thus has the apparent advantage of unifying what may initially appear to be disparate states, such as pain, injury, and death, by allowing them to be grouped under the common criterion of states of the body or mind that people disvalue as evils.

A weakness in this approach to the normative analysis of disease is that it makes the status of disease dependent upon the willingness of the members of society to recognize a particular state of affairs as evil. Those with hypertension may not feel any loss of capacity, but the physician operating with a nonnormative sense of proper physiological functioning can say that disease is present even if the patient would not. Similarly, a culture that has no written traditions may be unaware and unconcerned about the presence of dyslexia in some of its members. But a psychologist studying the group may be aware that a nondisvalued abnormal condition is present and may wish to intervene to modify the problem in order to allow a dyslexic member of the group to learn to read should he or she move into another society.

Normativism versus Nonnormativism —What Is Really at Issue?

The debate about the role played by values in the definition of health and disease may appear to be nothing more than an abstract philosophical controversy having few if any consequences for either the clinical practice of health care or the formulation of health policy. However, once the underlying concerns motivating the debate are made clear, it can readily be seen that what is at issue are understandings about the aims of medicine and the scientific status of its practices.

Normativists and nonnormativists are equally concerned with supplying a definition of health and disease that is capable of roughly capturing our intuitions about what ought to be classified as a disease and who ought to be viewed as healthy. But those offering definitions are also concerned with providing a definition that can help classify ambiguous states of the body or mind or resolve uncertainty where disagreements exist as to the proper classification of a condition as a matter of health or disease.

Aside from the aesthetic appeal of living in a world where conceptual matters admit of neat and tidy resolutions, there are important reasons for undertaking these definitional efforts. Unless medicine and the other health care professions use definitions of disease and health that are clear and univocal, there is a grave danger that uncertainties will exist on the part of both health care providers and patients as to the aims, goals, expectations, and hopes they bring to medical encounters. If health and disease are nothing more than socially determined, culturally mediated, or individually subjective concepts, then some fear that there will be little possibility of either placing medicine on a firm scientific footing or of finding consensus among experts and patients as to the proper limits of medical concern.

If, on one hand, one doubts that judgments of value are in any way objective, then the presence of values in the definition of health and disease will make it impossible for health care and medical science to rest upon an objective and universal foundation. If, on the other hand, value judgments are seen as amenable to objective reasoned argument, then their presence in the definitions of health and disease will do nothing to undermine the objectivity or scientific prospects of medicine and health care.

Why should it be presumed that values and objectivity or even consensus are incompatible? If it is possible to obtain agreement among rational human beings that some states of the body or mind are valuable and desirable while others are not, then it ought to be possible to accord an explicit role to values in the definition of disease and health without sacrificing objectivity, precision, or universality. Since there would seem to be no lack of agreement among patients and health care providers that under ordinary circumstances life is preferable to death, ability is preferable to disability, and pleasure more desirable than pain, then those committed to normativism would appear to have at least some grounds for optimism that an objective foundation can be built upon which to rest value-laden definitions of both health and disease. While this may be harder to do for some conditions or states than others—i.e., is it better to be born with large or small breasts or penis?—it seems that the goods and evils that bring people into the health care system and motivate others to want to practice the art and science of health care form at least a rough area within which consensus can be reached about what is good and what is bad and therefore what is health and what is disease.

The controversy over normativism and nonnormativism that has occupied center stage in recent thinking about health, illness, and disease may be more illusory than real. If the motivation for the controversy is the fear over the subjective nature of values, then it may be possible to defuse the debate by noting that it is possible to achieve agreement and consensus about values as well as facts. If this position is acceptable, then it may be possible to define disease as disvalued dysfunction where dysfunction is defined in terms of both human goals and the design of the human body (and mind, to the extent to which this can be known). Health would become valued forms of functioning, optimal or maximum, in certain systems or tissues. The extent to which values are seen as a source of difficulty for objectivity in the definition of health and disease will determine the degree to which one's sympathies lie in the normativist or nonnormativist camp.

sixteen

Curing What Ails the Medical Model

Rising Costs and Diminishing Access —An Intractable Dilemma?

A GREAT DEAL OF FERMENT IS EVIDENT in current discussions of the future of health care in the United States. Providers, seeing their autonomy restricted by a growing torrent of regulations, paperwork, and bureaucratic demands, are complaining vociferously about the red tape that is an all-too-familiar feature of health care in the United States. Managed care companies are pulling billions of dollars out of health care and putting it into their own pockets as the price of their attending to the bottom line.

Despite the high cost of health care, many Americans still lack adequate access to necessary services. Roughly thirty million Americans have no health insurance. Tens of millions of Americans dread the prospect of a prolonged hospitalization or extended stay in a nursing home, knowing they lack adequate medical insurance. The United States is spending more on health care than any other comparable nation but is receiving less coverage of its citizens.

The problems facing those concerned about the provision of health care or access to it do not end with a recounting of inadequacies in the current jumble of delivery and financing approaches to paying for health care. New technologies, both diagnostic and therapeutic, continue to pour out of the medical research cornucopia at a rapid rate. Some experts (Aaron and Schwartz, 1984; Schwartz, 1989) lay the blame for the high cost of health care squarely on the doorstep of biomedical research. Success in the discovery and dissemination of medical technologies, progress funded in large measure by public monies administered through the National Institutes of Health, has brought in its wake all manner of burdensome fiscal consequences. Health policymakers in the United States must struggle to solve an ironic problem—how to ensure equitable and affordable access to the fruits of the many successes achieved through publicly funded biomedical research. It is hard to refuse the latest and the best medical technology to anyone when that technology has emerged from a system of publicly financed research.

One early public policy strategy for coping with the problem of success was to make the benefits of technology available to all in need. In 1972, the End Stage Renal Disease Program (ESRD Program) was added to Medicare. The program was explicitly created to obviate the need for doctors to make hard choices about whom to dialyze when faced with the prospect of more persons dying from renal failure than could be treated given the available supply of dialysis machines. The program initially was intended to help 20,000 Americans suffering renal failure overcome the hurdles of high costs and a shortage of machines to gain access to a life-extending treatment. The estimates were that making dialysis and kidney transplants available to all would come at a price of $220 million. Within two decades the federal government was spending over $4 billion to provide various forms of renal substitution therapy to more than 100,000 Americans with failed kidneys, including the very old, the very young, and the terminally ill.

This early experience with solving the problem of technological success by lowering the "green screen" to allow universal access to a necessary health care service has occupied a central place in the consciousness of health policymakers in the United States. The explosive cost of the ESRD program for those with a relatively rare form of life-threatening organ failure bred a generation of cynics where the public financing of health care in the United States is concerned. The costly attempt to avoid the need to ration access to care by providing universal access to all who needed a high-tech solution cast an exceedingly long shadow across subsequent efforts to provide universal health care coverage for all Americans.

Technology often is seen as the culprit responsible for the cost explosion in U.S. health care. Still, Americans have continued to believe in the power of technology to solve medical problems. The high cost of many technological interventions continues to distort the access Americans have to the benefits of technologies aimed at reversing the course of acute diseases or injuries.

Access to various forms of organ and tissue transplants, for example, is closely tied to the ability of those in need to demonstrate the ability to pay for these procedures (Caplan, 1989; Wilson, 1996). This is true even though the provision of the organs and tissues that are transplanted depends upon a system of procurement that is deeply rooted in a public policy of voluntary generosity and altruism (see chapter 10 in this volume; Caplan and Bayer, 1985; Caplan, 1986; Kluge, 1989; Caplan, 1992). Moreover, the ability to pay determines access to most forms of organ and tissue transplantation even though the public has supported the proliferation of transplant centers throughout the United States through a variety of direct and indirect subsidies for organ and tissue procurement agencies, hospitals, pharmaceutical companies, and medical training (Kluge, 1989).

Can Philosophy Cure Our Ailing Health Care System?

The fact that the flow of new inventions and innovations shows no sign of abating is leading many health policy experts and government officials to promulgate Cassandra-like warnings about the inevitability of rationing access to health care (Churchill, 1987; Kitzhaber, 1989; Lamm, 1985; Aaron and Schwartz, 1984) and the impending collapse of government programs for the poor and the elderly (Peterson, 1996). Proposals as to how to implement rationing range from suggestions that the elderly will have to be deliberately shut out of the health care system (Callahan, 1987) to calls for rationing by excluding those who are perceived as responsible for or causing their own medical problems (Menzel, 1983; Rodmell and Watt, 1986; Blank, 1987; Caplan, 1995a) through the choice of unhealthy lifestyles, dangerous occupations or imprudent conduct with respect to drugs, sex, or the operation of motor vehicles. As former Surgeon General C. Everett Koop has warned, there is a grave danger that our health care system will "replace forgiveness with retribution" when confronted with health problems that are seen as arising from self-inflicted harms of one sort or another.

Another line of response to the seemingly never-ending flow of expensive new technologies is to argue that the ability to pay should determine who does and does not have access to expensive forms of health care (Kitzhaber, 1989). Proponents of the marketplace argue that health care will and should be distributed as are most other goods in the United States—by price. The moral commitment to ensuring equal care for all regardless of the ability of the individual to pay exhibited in the creation of Medicaid and Medicare in the United States and in the creation of various national health insurance plans in other nations, such as Great Britain, Canada, the Federal Republic of Germany, Norway, and Sweden, is weakening in the face of rising costs on both sides of the Atlantic. Egalitarianism is foundering on the rocks of cost. A key reason for the collapse of the Clinton health care plan, voiced most notably by the yuppie TV commercial couple, Harry and Louise, who were omnipresent during the height of the debate, was the perception that the upper and middle classes would lose access to the latest and best forms of treatment as the price of securing coverage for the poor and underinsured.

What is perhaps most interesting about the inability of the United States to deal with the challenge of providing access to care for all while containing cost is that the true conflict between cost and access has yet to occur. True, today some Americans die because they cannot afford the cost of primary care or a bone marrow transplant. But these cases are still unusual and rare. This situation could change in the decades to come. The American population is graying, and that means significant increases in the demand for health care services. Since the elderly use the most health care and technology in today's system, the prospects for incredible levels of rationing loom as inevitable in the not-so-distant future.

One in nine Americans in 1980 was over age sixty-five. By 2030 the ratio will have grown to one in five (Rice and LaPlante, 1988). The fastest-growing segment of U.S. society is the group that is at the highest risk of needing public support for health care services as a result of chronic illness, disability, functional impairment, and loss of the ability to live independently (Rice and LaPlante, 1988). It is likely that as improvements in acute care technologies lead to further declines in mortality, the number of Americans who have disabilities or restrictions of some sort in their cognitive or functional abilities will increase.

The ranks of those with chronic disability and impairment will grow not only because Americans are living longer but also because acute care technologies can be used to rescue persons who once would have died from acute disease or trauma. Extremely premature babies who survive as a result of neonatal intensive care units, children who survive on respirators or dialysis, adults who survive traumatic injuries to the brain or spinal cord as a result of advances in neurosurgery and in emergency and intensive care, or those who have been severely burned and maimed as a result of accidents are often rescued from what would have been the fatal consequences of disease or injury. But they survive with chronic, irremediable conditions (Jennings, Callahan, and Caplan, 1988). The number of such persons is growing. Their care will add to the already burgeoning health care costs, which will increase the pressure to contain these costs.

This picture is admittedly bleak. Strange as it may seem, ethical analysis may afford an answer to this impending crisis.

What, it is reasonable to ask, can ethical analysis possibly contribute to this bubbling maelstrom of health policy debate? If anything is true, it would appear that the time for abstract, ethereal philosophizing is long since past in the context of the debate about health care. The quintessential American response to crisis is to stop talking and start acting. Philosophical rumination seems a luxury that ought not be tolerated, much less looked to for answers in the face of crisis. What is required, the experts say, is a combination of bold policy initiatives, dynamic leadership, and decisive actions, not more analysis.

Bioethics is relatively helpless in comparison with other fields and professions purveying fast solutions or quick fixes for the crisis in U.S. health care. Philosophical analysis is rarely grounded in anything even vaguely resembling quantification, and in matters where budgets and values conflict, victory almost always goes to those who can adduce algorithms, mathematical models, and formulae to clothe their agendas.

Nonetheless, the attitude that the time for careful reflection is past when faced with current and future crises is wrong on any number of counts. Advances in the ability of the health care system to rescue lives that would once have been lost to acute injury and disease highlight the fact that we have had relatively little discussion, much less systematic efforts, to obtain societal consensus about the aims and goals appropriate to health care when life might be prolonged but with severe impairments. Progress in the treatment of acute disease and success in affording longer lives to more Americans opens the door to key philosophical questions about the response, in terms of both health care and public policy, that is appropriate in the face of a rise in the incidence of chronic illness, disability, and impairment (Jennings, Callahan, and Caplan, 1988). Philosophizing about the goals appropriate to health care is not so much a luxury as it is a necessity forced upon us by our society's own success in treating a wide range of what were once acute, lethal diseases.

There is a grave danger that the discussion of the enormous costs of health care and the need to do something, anything, to rein them in will lead our nation to enact policies that are at best indifferent to the norms and values which historically have been viewed as necessary to guide the provision of health care and ground health policy (Priester, 1989; Daniels,

Light, and Caplan, 1996). The stakes are so enormously high where policy options such as publicly legitimated rationing are concerned that it is hardly a luxury to subject the health care system to ethical examination in terms of its aims, goals, and purposes before bitter policy medicine is prescribed. Abstruse philosophy is just what the doctor ordered for a health care system desperately in need of cures.

Odd as it may seem, some of the debates about whether and how to reorient the health care system of the United States do hinge upon the definitions that are given to the foundational concepts of biomedicine. Our view of what to do in the face of disease, impairment, and illness is very much a function of what we take these concepts to mean. Philosophers are often accused of being entranced by the meanings of words. That may be so, but in disputes over the future direction of health care, words and their meanings matter, for the means for reaching goals in health care are inevitably determined by what those goals are understood to mean.

If You Are Not Sick, Are You Healthy?

It is odd that few medical, nursing, or pharmacy textbooks spend much time discussing the aims or goals of professionals in these fields. The relative silence over these matters in most texts and courses is a result of the fact that the aim of medicine or nursing may seem patently obvious and thus not in need of examination.

Doctors and nurses fight disease and repair injury. That is what people who go into a health profession expect to do. Someone with a fractured tibia, emphysema, or claustrophobia does not need to converse with a philosopher to figure out what they want their health care provider to do. People who are injured or sick want help, and most Americans believe that those in the health professions have, through their training, skills, and technological equipment, the ability to provide it.

While combating disease and injury surely occupies center stage among the universally acknowledged aims of health care, other goals might be served as well. For example, are those in health care responsible for promoting or preserving health? If so, are they then responsible for treating any and all factors that may cause injury or disease, including poverty, the lack of housing, illiteracy, and poor sanitation? The debate about physician-assisted suicide hinges in part upon the understanding that people have of the aims and goals of medicine. Is medicine charged with relieving pain, controlling suffering, or simply doing whatever it is that patients request be done?

Medicine's goals can be seen as quite broad. I recall hearing Jack Geiger, a physician at the Sophie Davis Medical Center of the City University of New York, tell of the time he and other physicians who were working in the South in the early 1960s took it upon themselves to write prescriptions for food for poor people suffering from the effects of malnutrition. They saw their goal as helping people to be healthy, and food was what poor people in rural areas needed most. So they prescribed it. The constitution that created the World Health Organization speaks of health as a "state of complete physical, mental and social well-being" (World Health Organization, 1946). If that is what health is and medicine is supposed to aim at reaching that goal, then it will be exceedingly difficult to define any boundaries as to the scope and responsibilities of health professions and the health care system.

Even if it is presumed that it is clear what health care professionals ought to do in fighting illness and repairing injury, what does it mean to say that those who provide health care ought to preserve or promote health? It is not at all clear what health is.

If people are not sick or injured, are they healthy? Or is health a state of physical or mental functioning that goes beyond the absence of illness, injury, and defect (WHO, 1946)? Or to put the point another way, is health merely the absence of disease or is it a state with its own defining properties and characteristics? (See chapter 15.)

Some health care providers—psychoanalysts, cosmetic surgeons, massage therapists, sports medicine specialists, electrologists, dietitians, physical therapists, dermatologists, among others—sometimes engage in activities that have as their goal a substantive conception of health that goes beyond the absence of disease. Optimal functioning or structure is the goal of at least some of the interventions carried out in our health care system (see chapter 15).

Surely it is possible to detect differences in the health of those who are not diseased or sick. Marathon runners and philosophy professors rarely possess the same degree of aerobic health unless they are both runners and professors. Pediatricians and endocrinologists are trying to decide which children are short enough to merit the administration of growth hormone, suddenly made available through biotechnological engineering. The use of drugs to enhance stature is another example where disease amelioration is lapping over into health promotion.

It seems reasonable to view health and disease not as opposites but as complementary concepts. The term *health* has as its conceptual opposite *unhealthy*, while the conceptual opposite of *impairment* and *disease* is not *healthy* but *unimpaired* and *not diseased*. If these distinctions are embraced, it becomes possible to ask a basic question, one which, while of fundamental importance, is almost never asked in arguments about the future direction of U.S. health policy—who is responsible for health and who for disease? If health and disease are not conceptual opposites then it may be appropriate for some parts of the health care system to pursue one or the other but not both, or for the pursuit of health to be a goal that is assigned to persons who work outside the arena of treating disease and injury. If health and disease are conceptually distinct, then it is an open question for public policymakers to decide which is more worthy of social resources. If health and disease are seen as complementary, parallel concepts, it is reasonable to raise the question as to which groups, institutions, and professions are best suited to meet the aims of promoting health or combating disease.

The answer to the nature of the relationship that exists between health and disease requires an examination of the ways in which disease is defined. While such an examination is definitely a philosophical task, it is an inquiry with high stakes. For not only do answers to what ought to be done to promote and preserve health hinge on what we think the relationship is between health and disease; basic questions about who ought be involved in the treatment of disease and what sorts of skills and training they should have revolve around the answer that is given.

Normativism and Its Consequences

To label a state or condition as a disease is to permit intervention by medical personnel, to grant access to various forms of social benefits, to confer a degree of exculpation from social roles and moral expectations, and to provide a framework for prophylactic, ameliorative, curative, and rehabilitative strategies. This fact has hardly been lost on the members of certain groups whose physical condition or behavioral propensities have left them hovering near the borders of disease. Alcoholics, gamblers, drug addicts, obese persons, hyperactive and learning disabled children, those made sick while serving in the Gulf War, and other subpopulations have fought long and often heated battles to gain entry into the realm of disease. Others, such as homosexuals, have fought against the disease label (Kass, 1975; Nimz, 1989; Caplan, 1995).

Debates about what is or is not a disease and the evolution of professional medical opinion as to whether a particular state or behavior is or is not an instance of disease provide support for one prominent line of thought concerning the definition of disease—that disease is an inherently value-laden concept. Those who subscribe to the view that definitions of disease must necessarily invoke references to norms or values can be usefully described as normativists. Normativists believe that mere descriptions of the status of the body or mind or the functional output of an organ system say nothing about whether someone is sick, impaired, or diseased. The only way to transform a biological fact into a disease ascription is by assessing the biological fact in the light of functions, capacities, abilities and powers that are considered desirable or undesirable, useful or useless, good or bad.

Diseases, in the normativist view, do not wear their identities on their sleeves. What is a disease in one context or social setting may not be in another. The only way to know whether a particular state or behavior is an instance of disease is to know what it is that an individual or group values and disvalues (Sedgwick, 1973; Caplan, Engelhardt, and McCartney, 1981; Caplan, 1995).

If values are truly inextricable elements of any definition of disease, this conceptual fact has direct implications for contemporary debates concerning the future direction of health policy and rationing. The identification of disease states as targets for either therapy or prevention will depend upon the degree to which societal consensus exists about whether a particular state or condition is good or bad. The treatment of disease might involve the provision of therapy or rehabilitation to restore function or ameliorate impairment, but it could also involve an effort to shift social views as to the evaluation that lies behind labeling a particular condition as a disease. The cure for a disease may require changing social attitudes rather than readjusting physiological variables. Some would call being short a disease. And there are many studies showing that for men, being shorter than average can have disadvantages in the workplace. But the cure for this problem may involve changing attitudes about height rather than supplying growth hormone to kids with short parents.

The recognition that values play determinative roles in the classification of states and behaviors as diseases indicates that the locus of intervention in responding to or coping with disease can be quite broad, including social, economic, even moral interventions as well as pharmacological, nursing, and surgical responses. Normativists see the determination of disease or impairment as subject to the analysis of both professionals and individuals, since the values that determine well-being, unhappiness, or handicap are in the eye of the beholder and the professional.

There is, however, significant opposition to the view that disease is an inextricably value-laden concept. Some view disease as a statistical concept that indicates only abnormality or deviation from a widely recognized paradigm of what is normal or as any state that is far removed from what is the general average for the population. Others argue that disease can be defined without reference to values, since disease refers to those states or behaviors that place an organism at a biological disadvantage in terms of survival or reproduction (Boorse, 1987; Caplan, Engelhardt, McCartney, 1981).

Nonnormativism, if valid, also has direct and important repercussions for health policy and health planning. The scope and range of health care would be limited to those aspects of human life where sufficient knowledge exists concerning the functions of the human body or mind to form a baseline for the assessment of disease. Ignorance of the design of the human mind or body or of whether or not a particular behavior or trait is advantageous in terms of survival or reproduction would make it impossible to say whether something is disease or represents an impairment. The locus of health care interventions would be skewed toward the individual rather than efforts to change the environment, culture, or social values, as would be possible in a normativist view, since linking disease to dysfunction encourages efforts to restore function directly rather than indirectly. Biology and organic functioning are the centerpieces of intervention in a nonnormativist view of disease.

Authority over disease would lie mainly in the hands of those able to make functional analyses relative to their understanding of ideal functional design of human beings. Judgments of illness, disease, and impairment would fall to professionals, since it is quite possible on the nonnormativist view of disease for persons to be sick but to feel quite well. Hypertension or incipient diabetes represent examples of diseases where only a functional analysis can reveal the presence of a problem that would otherwise not be recognized by someone without the appropriate education and training.

Nonnormativism is the view that has dominated among health care professionals and indeed among health policymakers during the latter half of the twentieth century. When doctors treat disease they do so in the belief that their goal is to restore dysfunction. The emphasis on the normal and the abnormal in medical diagnosis and rehabilitation is a reflection of the prominence of nonnormativism as the dominant philosophy of medicine. And the belief that the goal of medical research is to find cures for diseases, the belief that dominates much of the funding for health care in the United States, reflects an implicit nonnormativism concerning the nature of disease.

The Demedicalization of Chronic
Illness and Disability

Today's policy debates about health care are rife with confrontation: The old squaring off against the young to compete for increasingly scarce health care dollars. Doctors battling administrators so as to preserve their professional integrity in the provision of care. The needs of the acutely ill weighed in the social balance against the problems of those with chronic ailments and disabilities. Long-term care versus acute, exotic rescue efforts versus prevention, the needs of the few for enormous resources versus the needs of the many for small expenditures—the list of conflict goes on and on.

There can be no doubt that the resolution of some of these conflicts will require that hard choices be made. Some will not get the health care they want or need. But triage and rationing may not be the only answer to balancing the competing needs of the members of society. Part of the answer is to see the needs for services of many members of the population for what they are—the need for housing, social support, recreation, transportation, and security, not health care. One of the reasons our health care budget is out of control is that most of the services for the chronically ill, the disabled, the impaired, and the frail wind up on the health care ledger. They do not belong there. They belong on other budgets having to do with housing, transportation, crime, and other aspects of the quality of life. By medicalizing problems of daily living and turning them into challenges that can be met only by doctors and nurses, by hospitals and nursing homes, we not only risk driving our society into bankruptcy but also fail to provide the kind of services that people who are weak, frail, disabled, or vulnerable often require.

The Demedicalization of
Disability and Dying

The solution to the dilemma of how to afford the costs of high technology and modern medicine is, strange as it may seem, to limit the costs for those services to those who are truly diseased. Health promotion and the provision of services to the disabled and the terminally ill often do not satisfy the goals of modern acute care medicine. By forcing them into this arena we not only require individuals to be "medicalized" but we also ensure that those providing them services are poorly trained and ill prepared to do so.

The lesson of hospice is especially instructive in this regard. Dying has become an event that occurs in intensive care units for hundreds of thousands of Americans. There is no reason that this should be so. The irreversibly dying do not need intensive care. They need spiritual support, palliative care, familiar surroundings, and a peaceful environment. ICUs provide little of this. The staffs who work there are notoriously inept at handling these problems. It was only when some of those who worked with the dying rebelled and began to offer supportive care in the form of hospice that some Americans were able to escape a place most would never choose to die.

The demedicalization of dying that hospice represents is precisely the kind of recalibration that will lead to a resolution of our impending health care cost crisis. In many cases we do not have to force persons to forgo treatment or go without high-tech care; we simply need to make sure that they are either receiving appropriate services provided by appropriate (and almost always cheaper) care givers or that they get what they need outside the medical model.

If one listens carefully to competent residents of nursing homes (see Kane and Caplan, 1992, 1993) or the chronically ill and disabled, it quickly becomes evident that they do not see themselves as sick or diseased. And they do not wish others to see them that way either. The key to meeting their needs is not to create better training programs for physicians, to build more teaching nursing homes, or to place more emphasis on health promotion in our medical schools. These are places where the battles against acute disease and life-threatening injury are fought and should be recognized as such. The key is to create options and alternatives such as hospice and home care services like meals on wheels that allow persons to retain both autonomy and dignity without forcing them into a disease classification that then puts them in the maelstrom of an acute health care system that does not meet their needs. If we can change our understanding of who is sick and who is diseased, then the mission of keeping people healthy and supporting those who are impaired can be handed to those properly prepared to carry it out in appropriate settings at affordable costs.

seventeen

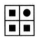

If Gene Therapy Is the Cure, What's the Disease?

Do Those Seeking to Cure Genetic Diseases Know What They Are Doing?

WHY HASN'T THERE BEEN MORE DISCUSSION of the aims and goals of those working on the mapping and sequences of the human genome in terms of the treatment of disease? Those who are actually engaged in mapping and sequencing the human genome or the genomes of other organisms often are not motivated by a particular practical goal or application. Despite all the hand wringing that has accompanied the evolution of the genome project, as well as the promises of therapeutic benefits that it will produce, many of those involved are simply interested in understanding the composition of the genome, its infrastructure or anatomy. Basic researchers have fewer reasons than clinical researchers to struggle to clarify the conceptual foundations of health, disease, and normalcy, and they will of necessity control the direction of the human genome project for many years to come.

In fact, those who are teasing out the secrets of the human genome have a positive disincentive to participate or encourage inquiries about the application of new knowledge in this area. If uncertainty about what to do with new knowledge in the realm of genetics is a cause for concern in some quarters, then those who want to proceed quickly with mapping the genome might find it prudent to simply deny that any application of new knowledge in genetics is imminent or to promise to forebear from any controversial applications of this knowledge.

Promising to avoid doing anything that will grossly offend societal mores is the simplest strategy if one's aim is not applying new knowledge but merely being allowed to proceed to acquire it. Some involved in the genome project have tried to defuse worries about the thorny issues of what constitutes health, what are the boundaries of normality, and what justifies referring to a particular genetic state as a disease by self-imposed restrictions upon the application of new knowledge concerning the genome. The clearest example of this prophylactic strategy is the promise that germline gene therapy will not be done (Walters, 1986; Anderson, 1989; Hall, 1990; McGee, 1997). The messy problem of how to fit new knowledge about heredity into existing categories of disease, normality, and health can perhaps be forestalled by arguing that the sole therapeutic goal of the human genome project is somatic genetic therapy for clear-cut instances of human disease (Anderson, 1989).

What Is Disease?

The easiest way to start an examination of how new knowledge of the human genome will influence how we ought to understand the goals of health care is by asking what it is today that doctors, nurses, psychologists, physical therapists, and the myriad other professionals who work in health care are supposed to do. The most obvious and commonsensical answer is that they are to combat disease. While many other goals might be and have been added, ranging from screening for eligibility for government benefits to certifying persons as fit to play sports or serve in the military, the fight against disease occupies center stage in what people expect health care providers to do. So if it is possible to become clearer about what disease is, then it may be possible to have a better understanding of the boundaries of what is and is not licit with respect to the application of new knowledge arising from the human genome project.

Two major points of contention are evident in writings that discuss the meaning of the concept of disease (Caplan et al., 1981; Caplan, 1989a; Scadding, 1996; and see this volume, chapters 15 and 16). One major source of disagreement concerns the role played by the determination of normality in the identification of disease. The other concerns the role played by values in the definition of disease.

Many physicians and nurses equate difference with disease or at least with a reason for suspicion that disease may exist. To put the point another way, abnormality is often viewed with suspicion either because it is seen as disease or because it is seen as symptomatic of an underlying state of disease. As E. A. Murphy cogently observed two decades ago in *The Logic of Medicine:* "The clinician has tended to regard the disease as that state in which the limits of the normal have been transgressed" (Murphy, 1976, 122). For example, many physicians and public health experts believe that blood pressure readings that vary from what is considered typical or normal for specific age groups within the population are in themselves indicative of disease. For physicians in the United States, variations skewed toward high numbers are disturbing. For German physicians, both high and low numbers are equally likely to be diagnosed as disease and therefore as sufficient to merit medical intervention. Similarly, variations even of a modest sort with respect to height, weight, attention span, sperm production, or blood cholesterol levels may trigger disease labels and consequent efforts at therapy.

Critics of what can be called the disease-as-abnormality approach point out that there is nothing inherent in difference that makes a particular biological, chemical, or mental state a disease. Moreover, since variation is an omnipresent feature in human beings, it is especially odd to argue that extremes of variation are somehow indicative of disease. If there is nothing at all unnatural about variation, then abnormality cannot in itself be equated with disease. Indeed, critics of the view that equates difference with disease note that throughout the history of medicine this equation has led to the classification of differences with respect to race, gender, and ethnicity as diseases, a classification that in turn has been the basis for unfair and even harmful interventions against persons suffering from nothing more than a darker skin color or the presence of ovaries (Gamble, 1991).

Those who are skeptical of the equation of disease with abnormality make two points worth pondering in the context of new knowledge about human heredity. First, simply labeling abnormality or difference as disease is of necessity the imposition of a value judgment on a physical or mental state that does not wear its disease status on its sleeve. Second, abnormality is not in itself bad. After all, those who are unusually smart, strong, fast, or prolific are not classified as diseased. If abnormality is to be equated with disease, then at a minimum the abnormality must be associated with something that is disvalued and there must be some connection between the difference or abnormality and the dysfunction that is disvalued (Clouser, Culver, and Gert, 1981; also see chapter 16).

These criticisms of the equation of abnormality and disease raise another major point of contention in defining the concepts of health and disease: whether it is possible to do so without reference to values. For if values must be used to decide whether a particular abnormality or difference is indicative of disease, then many worry that the entire process of defining health and disease must be subjective and especially vulnerable to political or social influences (Caplan, 1995a). If disease refers to abnormal states, either mental or physical, that are disvalued, then the appearance of values seems to some to make the prospects grim for objectivity or consensus about what states are or are not healthy or diseased. Subjectivity and a lack of consensus could bode especially ill for the uses to which new knowledge of human heredity might be put, since applications might be controlled by the powerful or the economically privileged to advance their own values.

Some believe that values need not be invoked in defining health or disease. Those who espouse nonnormativism, the view that the definition of disease need not involve any invocation of values (Boorse, 1975, 1976, 1987; Kendall, 1975; King, 1984; Scadding, 1967, 1996) usually invoke some notion of natural function or design to ground the definition of disease.

Nonnormativists doubt that values must enter into the assessments of organ function and behavior. For example, if a cardiologist says that the function of the heart is to pump blood or a renal physiologist claims that the function of the kidney is to cleanse the blood of impurities, it is not because they hold certain values about hearts or kidneys. Rather, based upon both functional and evolutionary analysis, it is possible to arrive at an understanding of what it is that the organs are supposed to do. By removing both kidneys or seeing what happens if the heart is damaged, it is possible to ascertain the functions of these organs. Therefore, nonnormativists argue, it is possible to use concepts such as cardiac or renal disease without invoking any sort of value judgments as to whether it is good that hearts beat or commendable that kidneys filter the blood.

Normativists argue that the concept of disease is inherently and inextricably value laden. They believe that functional analysis by itself cannot reveal whether a particular state of the body or mind is indicative of disease (Clouser, Culver, and Gert, 1981; Engelhardt, 1986; Fabrega, 1972; Goosens, 1980; Margolis, 1976; Pellegrino and Thomasma, 1988; Reznek, 1987; Sedgwick, 1973). For example, the fact that someone is nearsighted or farsighted may or may not be indicative of disease or disability. It depends whether one is going to spend one's day in the library, in the operating room, or hunting on the savanna.

Normativists almost always subscribe to the view that assessments of health and disease are value laden and that as a result they are inherently subjective, not objective (Fabrega, 1972; Sedgwick, 1973; Engelhardt, 1986). However, the link between the presence of values and the threat of subjectivity is open to question. The presence of values may make the definition of disease or health suspect in terms of its objectivity. But the existence of values in the assessment of health and disease does not mean that it is impossible to reach consensus about the definition of disease in spite of the fact that values play a role in the definition (Clouser, Culver, and Gert, 1981; Flew, 1983; Caplan, 1989a; Reznek, 1987).

Finding a Middle Ground

Equating normality with health and abnormality with disease as ways of defining these key concepts seems open to devastating conceptual and empirical problems. The view that what is different is in and of itself disease simply does not square with ordinary experience. Many differences are viewed as desirable or beneficial. Difference may be a cause for inquiry into whether a particular state is indicative of health or disease, but it is not in itself sufficient as a basis for deciding whether abnormality or variation represents health or disease in an individual or group. This is especially true for genetic differences, where it is already known that wide variations exist in terms of the genetic makeup of individuals that are not in any way manifest in their overt features, traits, or behaviors. Difference in and of itself does not always make a difference.

However, it does seem that the definition of disease and health is closely tied to those differences or abnormalities that are disvalued by the individual or group. If a particular trait, behavior, or physical structure is seen as causing impairment, dysfunction, pain, or other disvalued states, then it is a prime candidate for categorization as a disease.

The problem with linking values and abnormalities is that not all states commonly recognized as diseases are necessarily indicative of difference or abnormality. Nor are all dysfunctions or impairments always disvalued. For example, every human being may at some time suffer from the common cold, acne, anxiety, or dental caries. The universality of these conditions does not make them any more palatable or any less disvalued. It is possible for a state to be typical, normal, common, or universal and nonetheless be sufficiently disvalued that it is classified by both lay persons and health care professionals as disease.

Not every dysfunctional or impaired state is disvalued. Those who do not wish to have children may rejoice to discover that they lack a uterus, have ovaries that are incapable of ovulation, or possess testes that cannot create sperm. Someone born with only one functioning kidney may remain entirely indifferent to and even unaware of this dysfunction. Not all dysfunctional states are necessarily disvalued, meaning that not every abnormal state can be viewed as a disease.

Nevertheless, there does appear to be a conceptual link between abnormality, dysfunction, and disvaluation. If we restrict the definition of disease to cover only those mental or physical states of human beings that are abnormal, dysfunctional, and disvalued, then we will be able to identify many of the diseases recognized within a group or in a society.

Two questions confront those who admit the tie between disvaluation and dysfunction. Is it possible to determine the existence of dysfunction without invoking value judgments? If not, does the presence of disvaluation as a key criterion of the definition of health and disease make these concepts so subjective as to be either useless or extremely vulnerable to abuse by those powerful enough or privileged enough to impose their personal values on others (Caplan et al., 1981; Engelhardt, 1986; see also chapter 15)?

XYY and Oculocutaneous Albinism: Are These Diseases?

There is no need to resolve the disputes about normality or the role of values in the definition of disease in order to see what the consequences of these disputes are for new knowledge that is arising and will continue to arise in the domain of human genetics. The stance that those in clinical genetics adopt toward assessing the significance of difference and abnormality at the level of the genome, the role of values in defining genetic disease, and the need to link genetic disease to dysfunction will play pivotal roles in what is done with the knowledge generated by ongoing work to map and sequence the genome.

The question of how disease is assessed in the realm of clinical genetics is not entirely a hypothetical one. After all, counselors and clinicians have been treating patients for genetic diseases for decades. It is instructive to see how they define disease and health in order to forecast how new knowledge about human heredity will be absorbed into clinical and counseling practices. Two forms of genetic abnormality illustrate how much uncertainty and confusion exist about the criteria that ought be used to define both disease and the proper application of the concepts of health and disease at the level of genetic difference and abnormality.

A few years ago, a woman at a large medical center was informed by a genetics counselor that the fetus she was carrying possessed an abnormal chromosome. The child had XYY syndrome—an extra Y chromosome. The mother and father had sought genetic testing since she was in an age group at somewhat higher risk for a different genetic condition, Down's syndrome. The information that the baby had a different chromosomal abnormality from the one that had concerned the parents came as a surprise. Subsequently, in counseling sessions, the mother and father were told that a few researchers had posited a connection between criminality and this chromosome abnormality. They were also told that some researchers believed there was also a link between this condition and tall physical stature and even severe acne. After talking about the situation with their family doctor and various friends the couple decided to abort the pregnancy. Is XYY syndrome a disease? If not, why were the parents told that it had been detected? And if it is, is it a disease that merits aborting a fetus with this condition?

OCA albinism is a disorder in which melanin is absent or decreased in the skin, hair, and eyes. Albinism actually refers to the presence of a group of autosomal recessive traits in which the enzyme necessary for melanin production, tyrosinase, is present or absent in varying degrees causing a fair degree of heterogeneity. Most forms of OCA albinism are associated with a distinctive set of complications (Abadi and Pascal, 1989). Tyrosine-negative albinism, which occurs at a rate of about one in every 34,000 births (Wyngaarden and Smith, 1988), is associated with extreme sensitivity to light (photophobia), nystagmus, severe impairment in visual acuity, and a greatly increased risk of squamous cell skin cancer.

The genes involved in OCA albinism have been mapped (Spritz et al., 1990). Prenatal diagnosis is already a possibility using fetoscopy to obtain samples of fetal skin or scalp hair around the sixteenth week of development in order to see if the follicles contain melanin, but the relatively low incidence of the condition and the costs involved mean that such testing is rarely done. It will not be long, however, before a routine test will be available to detect this genetic abnormality from any sample of fetal DNA. Unless albinism is a disease, however, why should anyone try to detect it, much less provide information about it to parents?

In light of discussions in this and previous chapters about the complexities involved in defining disease, it is evident that decisions about what makes a condition a disease have direct implications for what will be done with information about XYY syndrome or OCA albinism. If one subscribes to the disease-as-abnormality definition, then both conditions will constitute disease states and both ought to be reported as such to parents. If one believes that it is necessary to draw a connection between disease and dysfunction, then OCA albinism will certainly qualify as a disease, whereas in lieu of more evidence, XYY syndrome may not. And if one takes the position that to be a disease a state must be both dysfunctional and disvalued, then it is possible that neither XYY syndrome or OCA albinism qualifies as a disease.

My own view is that it is difficult to defend the decision to label either XYY syndrome or OCA albinism as a disease. The former is an abnormality, but there is not strong evidence to support the view that it causes or is associated with dysfunction. The latter is an abnormality that produces dysfunction, but the problems associated with the condition are readily amenable to various interventions and coping strategies. It seems accurate to say that a person with OCA albinism is not diseased but has an abnormality that causes some impairment.

It should be obvious that the decisions that are made regarding the application of the concepts of health and disease in the realm of genetics require explanation and justification. It should also be obvious that not everyone will arrive at the same conclusion about the classification of human genetic differences, since people hold different views about what it is that justifies classifying a trait or characteristic as a disease, an abnormality, or a healthy state. Serious consequences follow the determination of disease states. Those in clinical genetics who diagnose and treat genetic diseases must not invoke the oft-espoused desire to remain value neutral as a rationale or an excuse for avoiding the obligation to carefully think through the criteria that are now used or others that might be used in the future to classify genetic diversity and differences as indicative of health or disease.

Implications of Defining Disease for the Study of the Human Genome

The realization that there is a broad spectrum of opinion about what makes something a disease is troubling in speculating about the ways in which new knowledge about the human genome is likely to be analyzed and classified. It is important to remember that much of the information that is likely to be acquired will reveal far more about the structure and composition of the genome than it will about its function. If we forget this, there is a grave danger that the disease-as-abnormality approach will find fertile ground in the realm of genetics in the future.

Some agreement must be reached about whether it is necessary to establish a link between genetic information and dysfunction or between dysfunction and disvaluation in order to establish the disease status of particular bits of the genome. Otherwise, increased screening and testing will reveal more and more differences and variations among our genomes, which will lead to an incoherent set of responses in terms of counseling, reproductive choices, and therapy. While consistency need not always be desirable, it seems morally incumbent on those who will be faced with the challenge of applying new knowledge about the genome to strive for some sort of professional and societal consensus as to how these questions ought to be answered.

For the present it seems clear that the first wave of new information about the human genome is likely to bear a fair amount of news about human differences that may have uncertain or unknown phenotypic consequences. Because clinical genetics is still in its infancy, it ought to proceed with great caution in labeling states or variations as abnormal, much less as diseases. For now, clinical genetics ought to restrict itself to the identification and assessment of only those genetic states that are known to be dysfunctional as well as different. It should discourage efforts to allow "fishing expeditions" to become part of prenatal, carrier, or workplace screening. And it should assert clearly that the central goal of human clinical genetics is the prevention or amelioration of disease, not the improvement of the genome. It is important to note that abjuring eugenics as a proper goal of clinical genetics is not the same thing as foregoing any effort to meddle or intervene with the genetics of reproductive cells.

Please Leave Us Alone: We Promise to Be Good!

Those who believe in the value of the human genome project, a group to which I belong, often try to calm fears about the misapplication of the knowledge the project intends to create by assuring all within earshot that their intentions are pure. This promise meets the concern of some of the harshest critics of the project (Rifkin, 1985a, 1985b).

A few of those who doubt that humankind knows what to do with more information about its own hereditary makeup or who simply believe that it is unnatural to mess around with genes sometimes try to arouse legislative or public concern by spinning scenarios in which man-animal chimeras slink out of the corridors of MIT, Cal Tech, Genentech, or Fort Dietrich to commit maniacal man-animal misdeeds against hapless humans. If such grim scenarios aren't scary enough, the occasional critic resorts to even more horrifying futuristic timeworms in which hordes of clones derived from the embryos of businessmen, sports stars, and politicians (no attempt is made to mitigate the horror) descend on an unsuspecting and defenseless world. The most hyperventilating form of such criticism consists of warnings to the effect that if the genome project is not stopped now, the result will inevitably be a planet teeming with millions of knockoff copies of Adolf Hitler, Genghis Khan, Saddam Hussein, Idi Amin, and Joseph Stalin.

Those who want the genome project to proceed apace are quite willing to promise never to xenograft a gene or to clone Hitler. If, by promising not to clone humans or even to perform germline interventions, the defenders of the genome project can allay the fears of their most strident and publicly visible critics, they are more than happy to do so (Anderson, 1989; Hall, 1990). This is especially true when the science fiction scenarios being spun are either scientifically impossible (cloning Hitler) or well beyond the reach of contemporary science (gene xenografting).

The greatest challenge to securing continuing funding for the genome project does not originate from concerns about privacy, confidentiality, or coercive genetic testing. It is eugenics, manipulating the human genome in order to improve or enhance the human species, that is the real source of worry. This is reflected in the content of the futuristic horror scenarios spun by the project's critics (McGee, 1997). It is also rooted in the historical reality of social policies based upon eugenics that led to the deaths of millions in this century (Proctor, 1988; Caplan, 1992c; Annas and Grodin, 1992).

Promising not to do anything that remotely hints of germline engineering in the service of eugenics is relatively easy for those connected with the genome project, since none of them believe that anyone is even remotely close to knowing how to alter the germlines of a human being, much less whether germline engineering will actually work. If the situation were different with respect to the practicality of germline interventions, then statements to the effect that germline intervention ought never to be attempted might be far more muted. Even without the prospect of imminent application, they should be.

The promise never to do germline engineering, invoked merely as an expedient to silence critics, is implausible because it rests on a flimsy moral foundation. Why shouldn't a couple concerned about passing along hemophilia or sickle cell disease hope that medicine can help alter their genomes so as to minimize their risks of doing so? Why shouldn't clinicians fervently want to undertake some forms of germline interventions so as to eliminate diseases such as Tay-Sachs, thalessemia, or Hurler's syndrome?

If it were possible to eliminate a lethal gene from the human population by germline alterations, is there any convincing moral reason why this should not be done? If those carrying a lethal gene request treatment so that they are able to reproduce without guilt or fear, ought not health care providers feel not reluctance but a duty to help them? If prevention and treatment of disease are the goals of human clinical genetics, then not only should germline therapy not be forsworn; it may be morally obligatory in cases where no somatic therapy is possible.

Should Germline Interventions Be Forsworn?

Some believe that any attempt at germline therapy is wrong, since it requires imposing the risk of harm on future generations, either by causing unanticipated side effects in unborn infants or by introducing dangerous genes into the gene pool. Future persons have no say in whether they consent to having risks imposed upon them. They, not their parents or ancestors, will suffer should attempts to manipulate the germline produce untoward results. Many bioethicists (Ramsey, 1970; Kass, 1975; Levine, 1986) believe and existing government policy in the United States, Germany, and other nations maintains that it is wrong to impose the risk of serious harm on those who cannot themselves consent. Newborns, very young children, the severely mentally ill and the severely mentally retarded should simply not be recruited as the subjects of pure research.

The other major reason for not undertaking germline interventions is that hereditary information which is of value not for the individual but for the species may be lost. If lethal or disabling genes are removed from a certain individual's gametes, it may be that benefits conferred on the population when these genes recombine with other, nonlethal genes will be lost.

A third argument against germline therapy is that no one would really want to use it for the purposes of eugenics. But this is patently false. Even putting aside Germany's thirty-year embrace of race hygiene and eugenics (Proctor, 1990), it is all too easy to find contemporary examples of governments and private organizations avidly and unashamedly pursuing eugenic goals. The government of Singapore instituted numerous eugenic policies during the 1980s, including a policy of providing financial incentives to "smart" people to have more babies (Chan, 1987). The California-based Repository for Germinal Choice, known more colloquially as the Nobel Prize sperm bank, has assigned itself the mission of seeking out and storing gametes from men selected for their scientific, athletic, or entrepreneurial acumen. Their sperm is made available for use by women of high intelligence for the express purpose of creating genetically superior children who can improve the long-term happiness and stability of human society.

Few protests have greeted those activities, whereas the hypothetical suggestion of someday directly modifying the genetic blueprint of a sperm or an egg has elicited great concern in many quarters. Granted, eugenics has been horribly abused in the past and may still result in terrible abuses today. But equating eugenics with germline therapy speaks simply of a confusion.

Should scientists or clinicians really promise never to try to eliminate or modify the genetic messages contained in a sperm or an egg if that message contains instructions that may cause sickle cell disease, Lesch-Nyhan syndrome, or retinoblastoma? The grim history of eugenically inspired social policy tells why it is important to protest and even prohibit the activity of the Nobel sperm bank or to vehemently criticize the birth incentive policies of Singapore (Duster, 1990). It does not provide an argument against allowing voluntary, therapeutic efforts using germline manipulations to prevent certain and grievous harm from befalling future persons.

There is no slope that leads inexorably from therapeutic germline interventions intended to benefit future persons to the creation of eugenically driven, genocidal social policies. Nazi eugenic policies were not aimed at benefiting individuals. The state or the Volk, not the individual, was the object of Nazi eugenic policy. A fascist ideology of public health, not a desire to provide individual therapy, was the driving force behind the Nazi medicalization of eugenics.

Worries about imposing harms on future persons without their consent or robbing the gene pool of the value of diversity are even less persuasive reasons for forswearing germline intervention. If the harms that will befall persons yet unborn are serious, even fatal, then it is far from self-evident that it would be wrong to try to prevent them, even if that means the imposition of possible risks for the child. The risks must be such that the child who is the involuntary subject of germline experimentation is at grave danger of being made worse off by the intervention. Some genetic diseases are so miserable and awful that at least some genetic interventions with the germline seem justifiable.

It is at best cruel to argue that some people must bear the burden of genetic disease in order to allow benefits to accrue to the group or species. At most, genetic diversity is an argument for creating a gamete bank to preserve diversity. It is hard to see why an unborn child has any obligation to preserve the genetic diversity of the species at the price of grave harm or certain death.

Forgoing efforts at germline engineering makes some political sense in the current climate of concern about the genome project. However, it makes no sense conceptually or ethically. The danger inherent in such stances is that they will result in the delay or loss of important benefits for persons who have impairments or diseases that might be amenable to germline engineering. The way to handle legitimate concerns about the dangers and potential for abuse of new knowledge generated by the genome is to forthrightly examine what are and are not appropriate goals for those who provide services and interventions in health care. There is nothing sacrosanct about the human genome. It is only our inability to openly and clearly define what constitutes disease in the domain of genetics that makes us feel that intervention with the germline is playing with moral fire. If it is eugenics we abhor, then it is eugenic goals that should be forsworn.

eighteen

What's Wrong with Eugenics?

The Repository for Germinal Choice

NESTLED BETWEEN TWO COMMERCIAL savings banks on a street in the small southern California city of Escondido is a very different type of bank. A small sign on the door reads "Repository for Germinal Choice." The people who use this bank have been carefully screened and selected. The Repository for Germinal Choice is in the business of trying to create better babies. It is a sperm bank on the cutting edge of eugenics.

Who might try to use the services of such a bank? Suppose you are a thirty-eight-year-old woman who has been thinking a lot lately about having a baby. You are worried about the number of ticks left on your biological clock. You are not married. The prospect of entering your "golden" years while your child is just getting out of high school is not especially appealing. You have a good job, can afford a child, and feel certain you would make a fine parent. Raising a child on your own looks like the answer. How to go about having one is the question.

You could do what some other women facing a similar problem have done. You could sleep with men without taking birth control precautions until you become pregnant. The prospect of recruiting strangers for sex, however, has little appeal. Having unprotected sex with strangers is just plain dangerous at a time when AIDS and other sexually transmitted diseases are at epidemic proportions. Trying to have a child without telling your sexual partner also strikes you as simply dishonest.

What about having sex with someone you know, someone to whom you can confide your intentions? The emotional complexities seem overwhelming. It would be wrong, you believe, not to admit that you are trying to have a baby to someone you know and care about. And having a baby with a man you know may create unwanted emotional entanglements between him and any child that results.

Adoption is another possibility. But waiting lists are long, and the odds of a single, older woman finding a child are not good. Moreover, while you are a bit ashamed to admit it to yourself, part of the reason you want a child goes beyond the desire to parent. You want a baby so that a bit of you will survive into the future.

If sex is out, maybe artificial insemination is the answer. You have read that many sperm banks do not accept single women. That may not be a big obstacle, however, since the technology for performing artificial insemination is not complicated. A simple turkey baster will get the job done. All that is really required is a source of sperm.

Some women have successfully used self-administered artificial insemination to bear children. The most daunting obstacles to success are timing the insemination attempt to coincide with ovulation and locating a man to provide the sperm. The options for solving the latter problem are finding a stranger willing to donate or, more realistically, a friend or nonblood relative.

A close friend or a sympathetic in-law might be an ideal choice, but there are possible emotional complications. If you use sperm from a man who knows that the child is his biological offspring as well as yours, there is always the danger that he may want to play a role in rearing the child. If he decides he does want to take on the social role of father, there is every reason to think that the law will support his claim. After all, whether you want him around or not, he will be the genetic father and, unless you marry, the only father the child has. Courts have generally been unwilling to totally break the ties between a newborn child and its genetic parents. In fact, should you change your mind and decide to involve him in parenting after the baby is born, courts would likely impose child support obligations upon him. If he insists on a parenting role, court-ordered visitation rights and even shared custody may well become a part of your life.

As you sort through the possible prospects and weigh the dangers of creating a child with someone whom you do not want to be a husband or father, another thought occurs to you. If you are going to use artificial insemination, why not find the best possible donor? As long as there is a choice, doesn't it make sense to use the sperm of someone who is smart, strong, talented, and handsome? After all, why shouldn't your child get the benefits of the best genetic blueprint available? Why should you settle for volunteers whose only qualifications are that they happen to be known to you and are willing?

Your decision to go it alone in having a child but to do so with an eye toward giving your baby the "best of everything," including genetic blueprint, might bring you to the Repository for Germinal Choice. For more than a decade the repository has sought to recruit sperm donors from the ranks of men of achievement in order to improve the genetic "stock" of future generations. The creator of the repository, optometrist Robert Graham, believes that the only way humanity can hope to meet the challenges of tomorrow is by breeding the right sort of leaders today. The repository is explicitly and proudly committed to eugenics as the appropriate normative foundation for childbearing. It tries to recruit a small, select group of men to serve as donors.

Originally the bank began by recruiting only winners of the Nobel Prize. Letters were sent to awardees, and when a man was willing, a storage container and a canister of liquid nitrogen were dispatched to obtain sperm for the bank. Nobel Prize winners are often older men; and after questions were raised about whether their age might be associated with damage to their genomes, the criteria for depositors were expanded to include younger scientists, business leaders, and athletes.

Once a donor's semen is obtained, it is screened for genetic disorders, defects, and diseases and then frozen. A book is prepared of the characteristics of the men whose sperm is stored at the bank, although specific names are not used. If the staff of the repository thinks that a woman seeking access to the bank has the right family history, IQ, and social achievements to satisfy them that a child might have the right hereditary "stuff" to solve the challenges of human life in the twenty-first century, then she qualifies to select a donor. Withdrawals from the sperm bank are kept anonymous. The donor will not know you have selected his sperm. It is up to you to tell your children how they were conceived. More than two hundred children have been conceived with the help of the repository, but it is not known how many are especially gifted or talented.

You may not come to the repository with eugenic visions in your mind. You may simply want to make sure your child gets the best possible start in life. Or you may decide that, other things being equal, you would rather choose the father's traits you deem might be advantageous for your baby. Your desire to select what, in your eyes, are desirable characteristics for your child may nonetheless complement the repository's desire to create a set of children with optimal biological endowments to solve the world's problems by leading the next generation.

The vision behind the repository is patently eugenic. The goal of the bank is to change the genetic makeup of future generations for the better. The goal of individuals who seek to create children with particular biological endowments is not obviously linked to the composition of the gene pool of the next generation. It is individual preference rather than benefit to the group, nation, or species that probably motivates the women who use the bank. Vanity or a desire to help others may motivate the male depositors. Still, choosing a gamete source from a sperm bank with an eye toward improving inherited characteristics constitutes a type of eugenics.

Individual versus Population Eugenics

In analyzing the ethics of the Repository for Germinal Choice or any similar eugenic program, a distinction should be made between efforts aimed at improving or enhancing the properties of groups and those aimed at allowing individuals to endow their children with desired traits. Attempting to choose the genetic makeup of a person or a couple's offspring with an eye toward specific features constitutes an individual eugenic goal. Efforts to improve the overall composition or makeup of the gene pool of a group constitute population eugenics.

Individual eugenics and population eugenics are conceptually distinct but may be pursued together. Those who, like Graham, want to pursue population eugenics may be able to do so either by allowing a group of those interested in individual genetic enhancement to pursue their individual goals or by recruiting like-minded people to pursue the goal of population eugenics. Individuals may contribute to the advancement of a eugenic goal unintentionally simply by pursuing their own individual choices.

The Repository for Germinal Choice has, since its inception, been treated in the media and academic circles as a crackpot sort of place, a fly-by-night facility run by a director who has bizarre dreams of creating a super race to solve the woes of the world. When the repository is not consigned to the nut file, its population eugenic goal leads some to dismiss it as a malevolent fringe, proto-Nazi organization.

Nazi ideologues did attempt to institute a form of population eugenics through coercive breeding programs. Racism was a cornerstone of Nazi ideology. Nazi judges and scientists ordered children killed who were thought to be disabled or genetically inferior to remove them as a threat to the genetic stock of the nation. Laws were enacted prohibiting marriages between those whom Nazi race hygiene theory held were likely to produce degenerate offspring. Steps to eliminate unfit or undesirable genes by prohibition of sexual relations, by restriction of marriage, and by sterilization and killing are all forms of negative population eugenics.

Conversely, the Nazis also did whatever they could to encourage those who satisfied Nazi racial ideals to have more children. The most extreme form of encouraging eugenic mating was the Lebensborn program, which gave money, medals, housing, and other rewards to persuade "ideal" mothers and fathers to have large numbers of children in order to create a super race of Aryan children. The provision of rewards, incentives, and benefits to encourage the increased representation of certain genes in the gene pool of future generations constitutes positive population eugenics.

Nazi race hygiene theories were false. There is no evidence to support the biological views of the inherent inferiority of races or the biological superiority of specific ethnic groups that underlay the eugenics efforts of the Third Reich. There is not even any firm basis for differentiating groups into races on the basis of genetics. The negative eugenics programs race hygiene spawned were not only patently unethical, since they were completely involuntary and coercive; they were also impractical and implausible. The Nazi drive to design future generations based on pseudoscience and racism led to concentration camps, forced sterilization, and genocide.

But the biological vision that motivates the Repository for Germinal Choice is not racist; it is not motivated by a theory of racial purity. Nor is it motivated by profit. The bank, which receives financial support from many private persons, does all that it can to remove financial obstacles for those it deems worthy of using its resources. Nor is the repository coercive. No one is forced to make deposits or to use the repository. Those who do freely choose to do so. The vision of the repository is elitist. The bank represents a distinct form of positive population eugenics, but it is a form of population eugenics that has little in common with the coercive and murderous policies of the Nazis. However, the eugenic optimism that fuels its operation does not square with what is known about heredity. In that regard it is a seriously flawed enterprise.

The Repository for Germinal Choice cannot deliver on its promise to create tomorrow's leaders. At most, using the sperm of Nobel Prize winners, corporate leaders, and great athletes only slightly increases the odds that intelligent, fit, and accomplished children will result. Human heredity is complicated. Traits such as intelligence, athletic ability, and personality are controlled by many genes, and these recombine somewhat randomly when egg and sperm meet. Every embryo, fetus, and child develops in a unique environment, so it is difficult to predict precisely what sorts of traits will be manifest in adults. Slight differences in biological makeup can make huge differences in physical and behavioral traits. As those with brothers and sisters know, having the same parents is no guarantee of similar personality traits, intellectual skills, or even physical similarities. So the repository seeks to bring about something that is currently beyond its reach in terms of what is known about human genetics.

Science and Eugenics

It will not be long, however, before science makes it possible to put eugenic aspirations into practice (Wilmut et al., 1997). The manipulation of gamete production to identify and eliminate unwanted traits and the ability to accurately insert genetic information directly into sperm or embryo are the subjects of investigation around the world. When these techniques are identified and refined, the chance to pick the biological endowments of our own offspring, to give them the "best" possible start in life, will have enormous appeal to many prospective parents.

The hope of using science and medicine to create children who get the best possible start in their lives is very different from the forced use of medical and scientific knowledge to solve society's perceived ills by creating biologically superior populations. There are those who would agree with Robert Graham that we owe it to future generations to maximize the genetic endowment of at least some of its yet-to-be-born members by showing some sensitivity to which genes are passed along from us to them. But the real advantage of new techniques such as the transplantation of sperm stem cells, embryo biopsy, and genetic testing of sperm and eggs is to fulfill the aspirations individual parents have for their children. Genetic enhancement in the future is much more likely to be the product of the norm that our children deserve the best than the imposition of a governmental mandate that we procreate in order to enhance the overall genetic makeup of our nation.

Although it is not easy to dismiss those who support using a sperm bank such as the repository as either eccentrics or Nazis, it is easy to dismiss the repository on the grounds that it cannot deliver on its promises. But to write the Repository for Germinal Choice off as just another example of stereotypical California fringe behavior would be a grave error. The aims of the repository and the motives of those who might choose to avail themselves of a place such as this if medicine could fulfill eugenic wishes confront us with the issue of the ethics of designing our own descendants. The day when we need to decide whether it is wrong to choose the traits of our children is not far off. When it arrives, we need to be clear about the ethical and public policy questions that will have to be faced with respect to making better babies.

For some, the historical abuses committed in this century in the name of eugenics, racial purity, and ethnic cleansing are sufficient grounds for prohibiting or banning any efforts at eugenics. However, if population eugenics is distinguished from individual eugenic motivations and it is agreed that parents do have a right if not a duty to maximize the well-being and happiness of their offspring, then it is not likely that the record of historical abuses carried out in the name of eugenics will rule out any efforts to incorporate genetic information into our procreative decisions.

If that is so, then what values should influence our ideas about human normality, perfection, and impairment? Can parents really be trusted to choose the characteristics of their children? Is the only reason that what Robert Graham and his associates want to do is ethically unacceptable is that they are holding out false hope because there is no guarantee artificial insemination by men selected for desired traits will produce these traits in their offspring? Making false promises to people is certainly wrong, but surely there are more fundamental issues involved in the ethics of intentionally designing "better" babies than false advertising.

Should We Pick the Traits of Our Children?
A Hypothetical Case

Suppose it becomes easier to achieve conception reliably outside the womb, making the analysis of the genetic makeup of embryos a simple task. Would there be any reason not to allow prospective mothers and fathers to select the biological endowments of their children? Before answering this question, think about the degree to which we currently make it possible for parents to obtain information about the genetic makeup of their unborn children in order to minimize the chance of having a child with a lethal or disabling medical problem. The hypothetical case of the Swansons may help shed light on how much a part of medicine individual negative eugenics has already become.

John and Maria Swanson had been trying to have a baby for a couple of years. Maria, who came from a large wealthy family, had completed her university studies in Central America. She had met John when she came back from Panama to study anthropology at a prestigious university in the Midwest. Maria discovered she was pregnant early in June 1996. She and her husband were ecstatic. They set about buying supplies and toys for the new baby and preparing the baby's room.

Maria scheduled her first prenatal exam at the University Health Clinic. Her obstetrician told her and John that since she was thirty-eight years old, she might want to consider prenatal diagnosis. He explained that because of her age there was a small risk, one in every 175 births, of her having a child with Down syndrome. There was also a risk for other serious chromosome abnormalities, roughly one in every 100 live births.

He suggested that one way to cope with these risks would be to undergo prenatal diagnosis. If the fetus was found to have a genetic problem, they might want to choose to have an abortion rather than to continue the pregnancy and deliver a child with a serious birth defect that they would then have to raise.

The last thing Maria and John had expected or wanted to hear from the doctor was a discussion about abortion. After all, this pregnancy was a dearly wanted one. But they not only wanted a child; they wanted a healthy child. Maria and John asked the doctor to tell them more about how prenatal diagnosis was done.

The doctor explained that prenatal diagnosis can be done in one of two ways. One type of procedure is called amniocentesis, which is performed around the sixteenth week of pregnancy. This involves passing a needle through the woman's abdomen into the uterus under ultrasound guidance to withdraw fluid from the amniotic sac surrounding the fetus. The fetal cells in the fluid are then grown and the chromosomes they contain examined. He told them that although the procedure is considered safe, about one in 200 women can have a miscarriage from complications such as premature labor, bleeding, or infection. Although needle injuries to the fetus had been reported, he said the likelihood of this happening was remote.

The second type of procedure for prenatal diagnosis is a relatively new test called chorionic villus sampling, or CVS. This involves obtaining a small amount of tissue from the placenta, the organ that feeds the fetus during pregnancy and appears as the afterbirth following the delivery of the infant. The major advantage of CVS is that it can be performed much earlier in pregnancy than amniocentesis, at around ten to twelve weeks, thereby offering the psychological benefit of the test results being available sooner in the pregnancy. Also, if the test results show a serious problem, the earlier an abortion is performed, the safer it is for the woman.

CVS can be performed either by a transabdominal approach or a transcervical approach, both using ultrasound guidance. The abdominal approach involves passing a catheter, a thin needle, through the canal of the cervix into the uterus and the placenta. Alternatively, a needle can be inserted through the woman's abdomen into the uterus and the placenta. Once the catheter is properly positioned, a piece of the placenta, called a villi, is withdrawn using suction from a syringe. The decision as to whether to use an abdominal or a cervical approach for CVS depends on how the uterus is positioned and what approach provides easiest access to the placenta. In other words, the Swansons' doctor said, it is a matter of the doctor's clinical judgment as to which approach would be easier and safer.

The doctor also told Maria and John that if they chose prenatal testing they could learn the sex of their fetus if they wanted to know.

Maria and John asked the doctor to repeat some of the details of the prenatal diagnostic options available to them. The doctor then left the room, and they talked it over and decided that they would have prenatal diagnosis. They both agreed that they would not want to have a child with a birth defect such as Down syndrome. Maria said she favored the chorionic villus test because it could be done earlier, early enough so that she would not feel so closely bonded to the baby if they decided to terminate the pregnancy.

The test was performed at eleven weeks of pregnancy. Everything went smoothly.

A few weeks later the doctor called and said he wanted Maria and John to come into the clinic right away to talk about the test results. An appointment was arranged for the next day. John and Maria, assuming as most parents would that a meeting on short notice meant bad news, spent most of the night talking about what they should do if their baby had Down syndrome. After much crying and soul searching they agreed that they would ask to have an abortion scheduled.

When they arrived for their meeting, the doctor got right to the point. The fetus did not have Down syndrome. But the test had revealed a different problem.

The analysis of the chromosomes in the cells taken from the placenta showed a balanced translocation between two of the chromosomes, numbers seven and eleven. The doctor reminded them that our chromosomes come in pairs. He then explained that a translocation meant there had been an exchange of chromosome material between one of the number seven chromosomes and one of the number eleven chromosomes. "OK, OK, but what does it mean, what does it mean?" John asked impatiently. The doctor said he did not know. He would have to test both John and Maria to get a look at their chromosomes. If either of them had the same translocation, there would be no problem for the fetus. But if neither had the same condition, there would be some risk of the baby's being born with a serious problem.

He asked Maria and John if they would consent to having their blood taken for the chromosome test. They agreed and samples were taken. A follow-up appointment was scheduled. As they were about to leave the office the doctor said he had one more question to ask. "Do you want to know the sex of the fetus?" John and Maria exchanged a quick glance. They had already decided they wanted to know, whatever the tests showed. Their baby was a girl.

The next few days were hard for John and Maria. They became more and more anxious and upset about not knowing whether their baby would be normal or not. They still had to wrestle with the question of terminating the pregnancy, a subject that filled them with dread. Maria persuaded John to drive to the university library to look up chromosome translocation. The articles and textbooks they found were hard to understand. Their anxiety only increased at their inability to know their baby's condition.

Three days after the diagnosis had been given, Maria and John found themselves back in the doctor's office. When the doctor came in they could barely stop themselves from jumping out of the chairs to insist he tell them what he knew. The doctor sat down and told them that the chromosome tests on both of them were completely normal. It took the Swansons a moment before they realized that this was not good news. The doctor reminded them that this meant that the chromosome problem had not been passed on from one of them but that it had occurred new in the fetus.

He said balanced translocations were very rare, occurring in about one in every 2,000 fetuses. He said the translocation could involve any chromosome pair but that only a few cases had been reported in the medical literature of an exchange between chromosomes seven and eleven.

"Seven, eleven, seven eleven." John could barely follow what the doctor was saying. Somehow all he could think about was that these numbers were supposed to be lucky but for some reason the roll of the dice for his little girl had come out against her.

The doctor said he really could not be sure what the translocation meant for their fetus. His best guess was that they faced a 5 to 10 percent chance of having a baby with a birth defect. John and Maria pressed—"What sort of defect, what sort of problem?"—but the doctor just shook his head. "The impact of translocations is almost unpredictable," he said. Their daughter could have problems that included mental retardation, a malformed heart or other vital organ, or skeletal abnormalities. On the other hand, there was a 90 to 95 percent chance the baby would be born healthy.

After some further discussion the doctor mentioned that they might want to call a couple of other experts in genetics to get their opinions. As soon as they got home they started calling. What they heard made them even more uncomfortable. One said they should not worry all that much. While there were risks involved, the odds favored a healthy birth. Another expert said that ultrasound testing could be performed later in the pregnancy to look for abnormalities of the heart, bones, and other organs. However, he could not totally reassure them that even if nothing was found on the ultrasound that the baby would not be born with problems.

They talked for days about what to do. John called his brother, who was horrified at the idea that John and Maria would knowingly bring a child into this world if the baby might have a serious birth defect. Maria was worried that even if the baby appeared normal at birth, the doctor had said there was still a risk of other problems developing later. John wondered whether he could ever treat his daughter as a normal kid knowing she had an abnormal genetic makeup.

Finally, after a week of agonizing they reached a decision. As painful as it was, especially in the light of how long they had waited for this baby, they did not want to risk bringing a child into the world who carried the burden of a serious birth defect. They decided to schedule an abortion within the week so that they could begin trying to have another child, a normal child, as quickly as possible. They called and told the clinic doctor of their decision. He said he was sorry they had to face such a difficult decision but did not try to change their minds. Two days later, at fourteen weeks of pregnancy, Maria Swanson had an abortion at the University Health Center.

When women seek sperm from the Repository for Germinal Choice, they are motivated by some view as to what are desirable traits that they wish their children to have. When the Swansons decided to end their pregnancy, they were motivated by a fear of an undesirable trait they did not wish to see their child possess. In both cases, parents are trying to make sure they do what is best for their child.

What should medicine do in the face of a strong desire most parents feel to bring their child into this world healthy? Is there any criterion or definition that would allow the sorting of human traits into desirable and undesirable categories? Even if such a classification could be done, is it part of medicine's professional responsibility to allow parents to pick and choose among the desirable and undesirable characteristics they wish their child to have?

Health, Disease, Disability, and the Aims of Medicine

Sometimes those interested in the ethics of reproductive choices based upon genetic considerations divide decisions based upon the desirability of traits into those that represent negative and positive eugenic concerns. Negative eugenics refers to choices or policies aimed at preventing genetic disease and disorders from being inherited. Positive eugenics describes efforts to improve or enhance the traits in an offspring or members of future generations. Even if the prospect of population eugenics is rejected as morally intolerable, is there still a moral case for permitting individuals such as the Swansons to use genetic knowledge for reasons having to do with negative eugenics? And if the case can be made for allowing negative eugenic concerns to influence and guide reproductive choices, can a parallel case be made for positive eugenic considerations?

To some extent the answers to this question revolve around the values that parents bring to the act of reproduction. But those in the practice of medicine also have influence over the kinds of concerns that are deemed appropriate on the part of patients seeking genetic information to guide their reproductive choices.

When most people think about health they think about it as referring to the absence of illness or disease. If you are not sick, then you are healthy. But this way of thinking about health, about what is normal and abnormal, is a little confusing. It is possible to be free of disease and still not be seen by others as healthy. You can be out of shape, nervous, on edge, or lacking in self-confidence, have no stamina, feel awkward, and still, on the view that the absence of disease constitutes health, be considered healthy. But that seems to stretch the meaning of health to include a bit too much. Health is not simply the absence of disease and dysfunction (chapter 15).

Health means something more. Health refers to a state in which persons are flourishing, in which bodies and minds are working not at adequate levels but at optimal levels. Health makes essential reference to a concept of optimizing, not merely reaching, some level of minimal functioning.

If it is true that health refers to optimizing the functions of our bodies and minds, then it is easy to see why health is such an elusive goal. Health is an ideal, not an average or a minimal threshold. When parents say they want a healthy child, they may well only mean that they want their child not to be sick, meaning to be disease free or able to function without serious impairments or disorders. But they may mean that they want a child who enjoys the best possible physical and mental functioning, a child who functions at optimal, perfect levels. This is precisely the sort of wish, the pursuit of perfection, that leads some men and women to want to use the services of the Repository for Germinal Choice. It could have been the sort of concern that led the Swansons to terminate their pregnancy when they found out that a translocation was present.

The desire for health, in the full sense of the concept, is behind parental decisions to place their child in the elite nursery school, the expensive private high school, the tennis camp, or special music or art classes. These institutions are valued not because they prevent disease or dysfunction. They are valued because many parents see them as the means to inculcating the best possible skills and abilities in their children. They are valued as a part of health, not as a means of avoiding disease.

How might the desire for health have played a role in the Swansons' decision to terminate their pregnancy when told a chromosome translocation was present in their fetus? The Swansons may have felt that having a child who was at risk of disorder was not in their child's best interest. They may have felt it would be morally wrong to bring a child with a serious birth defect into the world, since it would be wrong to saddle a child with a serious disability. But more may have been involved in their decision than a concern to avoid disease. They may have wanted a child who had a chance of reaching their view of what constitutes health, who could strive to achieve ideal or optimal mental and physical functioning.

The Perfect Child

Assume that those who seek out the services of a place such as the Repository for Germinal Choice want the healthiest possible offspring. Assume that what drove the Swansons to decide to end their pregnancy was their desire to pursue perfection in the attributes of their baby. Is there anything morally wrong with pursuing perfection as the goal of reproduction? What moral principles are violated by the desire to design one's children so they are as perfect as possible?

Arguments that are commonly made against the morality of trying to design perfect children fall roughly into three categories. One set of arguments is that coercion or a lack of choice on the part of parents in the choice of the traits of their children or in any area of reproductive choice is unacceptable. Thus the Nazi dream of perfecting a super race of perfect Aryans by eliminating the unfit, the handicapped, and those seen as genetically inferior is ethically repugnant because the government forcibly imposes its vision of perfection by force, sterilization, or murder. In the case of the Nazis their desire to increase the health of future generations was tied to the killing of those identified as less than perfect, along with coercive marriage and breeding for those believed to have desirable traits.

Some who find the pursuit of perfection objectionable on moral grounds are worried about more than coercion. They note that it is simply not clear which traits or attributes are properly perceived as perfect or optimal. The decision about what trait or behavior is good or healthy depends upon the environment and circumstances that a child will face. To pick traits, features, or attributes in the abstract is to simply reify prejudice into a strategy for the creation of optimality.

These arguments, while of grave concern in light of the history of abuse and genocide tragically manifest throughout this century, are not ultimately persuasive as the basis for prohibiting reproduction in the service of perfection. For the objections focus not on the desirability of perfection but on the means used to achieve this goal or uncertainty about what traits fulfill it.

Certainly it is morally objectionable to allow governments or institutions to compel or coerce persons into having children. The right to reproduce without interference from third parties is one of the fundamental freedoms recognized by international law and moral theories from a host of ethical traditions. It is also morally wrong to allow the state to impose its vision of the future by force. However, the goal of obtaining perfection or pursuing health with respect to reproduction is not made objectionable by these arguments. What is morally wrong is coercion or compulsion or arbitrariness with respect to reproductive decisions.

The Repository for Germinal Choice and genetics counseling programs at academic medical centers and private clinics make a special point of avoiding any hint of coercion or compulsion in their activities. It would seem that those who correctly find the reproductive policies of the Nazi regime in Germany during the Second World War, the government of South Africa prior to the creation of democracy in 1993, or the current population policies of China ethically abhorrent are repulsed more by the means than the goals involved in efforts to design future generations.

As for the objection that decisions about perfection are more a matter of taste and prejudice then they are value judgments rooted in solid empirical evidence, that is, in many instances, true. Decisions to produce tall children or those who have blue eyes are merely reflections of cultural or social preferences rather than objective properties having anything to do with disease or health. But there are certain traits, such as physical stamina, strength, speed, mathematical ability, dexterity, and acuity of vision, which are related to health in ways that command universal assent in almost any cultural or social setting imaginable. It would be hard to argue that a parent who wanted a child with better memory or greater physical dexterity was simply indulging his or her biases or prejudices. As long as no coercion or force is used to compel persons to make choices about their children that are in conformity with particular visions of what is good or bad, healthy or unhealthy, there would seem to be enough consensus about the relationship between certain physical and mental attributes and health to permit parents to choose certain traits, features, and capacities for their unborn children in the name of their health.

Moreover, it is not even necessary to achieve consensus about what is objectively good in order to allow parents to pursue a goal of genetic enhancement to improve the lot of their offspring. Parents might concede that their vision of perfection is to some degree subjective but still insist upon the right to pursue their own values. Since we accept this point of view with respect to child rearing, allowing parents to teach their children religious values, hobbies, and customs as they see fit, it would be difficult to reject it as overly subjective when matters turn to the selection of a genetic endowment for one's child.

Some maintain that efforts to genetically design children by picking embryos, by genetic engineering, or by controlling the use of gametes are morally wrong because they limit what the child can become. Imposing a parent's wishes on a child when a parent picks the height, aptitudes or appearance of the child is not something the child can do anything about.

To object to efforts to perfect kids on the basis of diminished malleability is not persuasive. Kids have no choice in their parents as it is, and it is hard to believe that it is more just to ask a child to accept the random luck of reproduction rather than sincere efforts to improve their lot. Given the latitude that parents have to shape and mold their children, restrictions on parental choice of biological makeup would cast doubt on the morality of the entire practice of parenting as it is now known in all contemporary societies.

A second set of objections commonly raised against trying to achieve perfection hinges on concerns about slippery slopes of various types. While not everyone who wants to use the Repository for Germinal Choice is a secret admirer or proponent of either negative or positive population eugenics as a matter of law or public policy, some observers worry that any opening of the door to permit parents to pick the traits of their children will lead inevitably to the government's forcing its vision of perfection upon anyone who wants to have children. But this argument has problems as well. It flies in the face of a number of facts about the pursuit of perfection in other areas of health care.

For many years, cosmetic surgeons, psychoanalysts, and sports medicine specialists have been plying their trades without any slope having developed in society to the effect that those with big noses or poor posture must visit specialists and have these traits altered. Some choose to avail themselves of these specialists in the pursuit of perfection. Most do not. If there is a slope from permitting individual choice of one's child's traits to limiting the choices available to parents, it is a slope that does not start with individual choice. And if there is a problem of a slope, then it must be shown why it is morally permissible to seek perfection after one is born but why such efforts would also be wrong if engaged in prenatally.

It is certainly true that twentieth-century history is full of instances of genocide, mass murder, and ethnic cleansing. These are, nevertheless, problems of politics, government, and ideology. There is nothing inherent in the decision to indulge one's preferences about the traits of one's child that is morally wrong as long as those preferences do nothing to hurt or impair the child. If there are slippery slope problems that confound the morality of eugenics, they lie in the flaws of politics, not in the desire to have a "better" baby.

A third set of objections to allowing eugenic desires to influence parenting is that it will lead to fundamental social inequalities. Allowing parental choice about the genetic makeup of their children may lead to the creation of a genetic "overclass" that has unfair advantages over those whose parents did not or could not afford to endow them with the right biological dispositions and traits. Or it may lead to too much homogenization in society where diversity and difference disappear in a rush to produce only perfect people, leaving anyone with the slightest disability or deficiency at a distinct disadvantage.

Equity and fairness are certainly important concepts in societies that are committed to the equality of opportunity for all citizens. However, a belief that everyone deserves a fair chance may mean that society must do what it can to ensure that the means to implementing eugenic choices are available to all who desire them. It may also mean that a strong obligation exists to compensate for any differences in biological endowment with special programs and educational opportunities. In a world that tolerates so much inequity in the circumstances under which children are brought into being, it would be hard to argue that there was something more offensive or more morally problematic about biological advantages as opposed to social and economic advantages. And in a world that gives large numbers of privileged persons the right to pursue the best education for their children in situations and contexts that may well produce homogeneity in the end results, it would also be difficult to argue that the pursuit of perfection or enhancement at the cost of homogeneity should be allowed when the intervention is environmental but not when it is biological.

There does not appear to be a persuasive or in principle ethical reason to close the Repository for Germinal Choice or to condemn families such as the Swansons for their decisions to end a pregnancy when a serious genetic disorder is found. While force and coercion, compulsion and threat, have no place in procreative choice, it is not so clear that it is any less ethical to allow parents to pick the eye color of their child or to create a fetus with a propensity for mathematics than it is to permit them to teach their child the values of a particular religion, to inculcate a love of sports by taking the child to games and exhibitions, or to require the child to play the piano.

If there is an argument to be made against eugenics, it would seem to be most persuasive against group or population eugenics. Efforts to shift the composition of the gene pool would seem to require or be more prone to slip toward the imposition of a vision by government or other powerful institutions. Insofar as coercion and force are absent and individual choice is allowed to hold sway, then, presuming fairness in access to the means of enhancing our offspring, it is hard to see what is wrong with trying to create better babies.

nineteen

Do Not Copy
without Permission

THE IMPACT OF THE ANNOUNCEMENT of the cloning of the first mammal—Dolly, a sheep made in Scotland by Dr. Ian Wilmut of the Roslin Institute and his colleagues (Wilmut et al., 1997)—and the first primates—two monkeys cloned at the Oregon Regional Primate Center by a team led by embryologist Don Wolf—was immediate and astounding. America began to hyperventilate over cloning.

Bizarre scenarios proliferated in the press, Congress, and lecture halls in which unscrupulous entrepreneurs used cloning to breed spare bodies for use as portable organ farms, animated a copy of dear old Uncle Fred whose six pack a day smoking habit took him from this mortal coil far too soon, or unleashed legions of subhuman cloned drones upon a hapless public (Carey, 1997; Specter and Kolata, 1997; Kendall, 1997). President Clinton moved quickly to ban federal funds for human cloning research and urged the private sector to do the same (Weiss, 1997). Calls rang out from Germany and other nations to ban all forms of cloning. Congress held so many hearings that the director of the National Institutes of Health, Harold Varmus, seemed to have little time for anything other than to condemn human cloning as morally repugnant (Seelye, 1997). Why was the reaction to the creation of mammalian clones so heated? And what does it say about the moral fears and concerns about the genetic revolution that bubbled forth once the cloning barrier was breached?

Reports of successful cloning using cells taken from adult organisms, in the case of the research in Scotland that produced Dolly the sheep, and success in copying monkey embryos in an Oregon primate center were important. They constituted major breakthroughs in genetic manipulation. The demonstration that it is possible to get genes from one creature to work when transplanted into the embryos of another was of monumental importance. Many scientists were skeptical that any technique could be found which would permit genes that had turned off in the course of adult development to turn back on. As Dolly showed, they were wrong. Put in the right environment—an embryo at a very early stage of development—adult genes would turn back on and guide the development of another creature as they had done when they first guided the construction of an adult organism.

Not only does cloning show that genes retain enormous capacity to transmit information over time; it also shows that under the right conditions the genetic instructions that guided the development of an entire complex creature can be tricked into doing the same thing again. This has obvious implications for understanding regulatory genetics, for diseases such as cancer which often have regulatory mistakes as a part of the disease process, and for understanding the course of normal development from embryo to fetus to adult. Cloning also holds the promise of unlocking many of the basic secrets of the ways in which nature and nurture interact to produce traits and behaviors. Using cloning, scientists can copy the same genome again and again and then examine the role played by various environmental factors in controlling the output of the same genetic information. Cloning also has obvious and attractive applications in veterinary medicine, in preserving endangered species, in commercial animal breeding, and in agriculture. But of course, while these were among the interests that the successful cloning of a monkey and a sheep excited in many scientists, including those who did the breakthrough work on cloning (Specter and Kolata, 1997), they had nothing to do with public interest in cloning or the hype which surrounded the announcement of the scientific work.

The appearance of cloned sheep and monkeys made it almost a lead-pipe cinch that cloning is something that could be done in humans. And it was human cloning that caused the eruption of ethical, political, and societal angst that greeted the appearance of Dolly.

The fact that a cloned sheep could run about in a pen in rural Scotland or some cloned monkeys loll about in a cage in Portland, Oregon, should not leave anyone wide awake nights wondering what ruthless totalitarian lunatic is going to send an army of heartless clones to attack Washington, D.C. Okay, bad example. You might fervently hope an army of clones attacks Washington or wonder whether, given the number of indistinguishable lawyers and lobbyists ambling about the nation's capital, the attack of the heartless clones is already well under way. Substitute Boston, Tucson, London, Toronto, Perth, Philadelphia, or some other locale that you love. The point is, worries about human cloning, while legitimate, must also be placed in perspective.

In order to produce Dolly, Scottish scientists had to start with nearly 300 sheep embryos. When they transferred adult genes into them, the overwhelming majority of the embryos died. Others developed abnormally or produced sick and defective sheep (Wilmut et al., 1997). A similar story on a smaller scale is true of the Oregon monkey experiments and other efforts to clone. It is still not known what impact on aging, growth, health, or behavior cloning will have on animals made using these techniques.

Current cloning technology is best understood as on a par with the flight of the first engine-powered airplane. Many argued that no one would ever fly in a machine. The Wright brothers proved them wrong. But it took many years, after the first short flight at Kitty Hawk, North Carolina, before the first safe, reliable, and practical aircraft was up in the air.

The same is true of cloning. The sheep in Scotland and the monkeys in Oregon represent first steps down what is a very long road. The techniques used are not only *not* safe to try in humans, they are not very effective or efficient for use in animals. Any technique that produces defective or sick sheep or monkeys is absolutely morally unacceptable for use in human beings.

While we might accept the creation of deformed sheep or a prematurely aged monkey as part of an experiment to demonstrate the feasibility of cloning, it would be morally incomprehensible to accept anything less than the tiniest of chances of creating a deformed or disabled human simply to demonstrate the feasibility of human cloning. (See chapter 3 for an analogous argument about the artificial heart.) Research involving children and the fetus has also required both a therapeutic intent on the part of the investigator and that minimal risk be posed to the fetal subject (Grodin and Glantz, 1994). Neither condition would be satisfied by an experiment aimed at testing the feasibility of human cloning.

If cloning a human being is so obviously immoral given the risk of deformity and death posed to the unconsenting human subject, why did so much moral anxiety arise in response to animal cloning? Pinpointing the causes of that anxiety will go a long way toward identifying the deep moral ambivalence that underlies public attitudes toward the entire genetic revolution. In reviewing the kinds of objections that appeared in the popular press, scholarly journals, and electronic roundtables that followed in the wake of the announcement of the cloning of Dolly (Caplan, 1997c; Carey, 1997; Maugh, 1997; Kendall, 1997; Sale, 1997; Schmickle, 1997), a number of key themes emerge: once unleashed, technology cannot be stopped or controlled; cloning is wrong because human beings are not wise enough to use it prudently; cloning threatens human dignity and individuality. Each of these themes illustrates very deep concerns within American and other societies about the genetic revolution. Rather than debate the merits of breeding clone armies or harvesting spare parts clones for tissues or blood, it is important to address these deeper concerns which fuel the more lurid and fantastic speculations about cloning.

Perhaps the most omnipresent fear that Americans and those in other nations had about the demonstration that cloning could be achieved in mammals was that there would now be no stopping the application of cloning to humans and eventually the abuse of cloning with humans for blatantly immoral purposes. This fear was best encapsulated by two common themes in many news-analysis and opinion columns—once the technological genie is out of the bottle it cannot be put back, and no technology that has ever been invented has ever been stopped by moral concerns (Caplan, 1997c; Carey, 1997; Kendall, 1997; Sale, 1997). Neither claim is true.

The first appearance of a new technological breakthrough does not thereby signal that the technology is of necessity beyond control or regulation. It will be years before today's cloning technology could reasonably be applied safely to the creation of human beings. If we do not want it to be, then it is up to us to engage in the moral, religious, and legal discussion that will make sure human cloning does not happen.

True, no one can stop a nut from grabbing a spare embryo at an infertility clinic and transplanting a set of adult genes into it to see if human cloning will work. And, true, curiosity as to whether cloning will work is a powerful psychological motivation in tempting scientists to want to try and find out. But these facts do not lead to an inevitable industry in, or routine application of, human cloning.

Making a human fetal clone in a basement or at the behest of a billionaire is the subject of tabloid headlines and soap operas, not science. Science to be science must be replicable and testable. The activities of crackpots and lunatics, while unfortunate, should certainly not lead anyone to despair about the ability to create and enforce laws. The fact that people rob banks does not lead us to abandon laws against theft and robbery. The fact that some people counterfeit money or pass bad checks does not lead society to abandon attempts to protect the integrity of national currencies. Nor should the threat of behavior on the fringe lead to the abandonment of reasonable means for controlling the pace of cloning technology.

If our society and others really think that it is an offense to human dignity to have people bred by design, if it is plainly morally offensive to let anyone create a human being just to have a place to get spare parts, or if we really do not want grieving parents trying to "restore" a lost child by using asexual reproduction to make a physical copy of the child's body, such activities can be brought to a grinding halt. How? Slap stiff penalties on human cloning, let researchers know that experiments on human cloning will not be published, pull all government and foundation support for human cloning research, teach scientists about their ethical responsibility to use cloning responsibly, and establish bans on using human cloning for commercial or financial gain. For all practical purposes human cloning will grind to a halt.

If the steps to control cloning are so easy to articulate, then why so much skepticism and despair that they would ever be enacted or enforced? Part of the despair about regulating cloning comes from the fact that worries about cloning are not new. They have long been present in American and British culture, for example, in movies such as Woody Allen's *Sleeper,* Lindsay Anderson's *O Lucky Man, The Boys from Brazil* (based on Ira Levin's novel), *Multiplicity* (with Michael Keaton), and Gene Roddenberry's *Star Trek* movies, notably *The Wrath of Khan,* and many television episodes in both the first and second series of programs which examine the use of cloning in humans and nonhumans. Cloning has long served as a focal point for society's worries about the power of genetic knowledge. All of these films and their television cousins tout the idea that science and technology must inevitably be our master. Human beings cannot, so the stories go, control the genetic technologies that they invent. Once cloning actually occurred, it very rapidly was asked to carry the burden of twenty-five years of fictional speculation about the moral dangers of genetics.

Fictional presentations raise important moral questions, but they do not prove that humans cannot control what they invent. The worry that the power to shape our genetic destiny will be misused or lead to societal disruption is real enough and surely has a base in the dismal facts of modern history, but worry is not the same as fate. The fears of the downside of genetic technology that haunt the silver screen and cable TV industry should not fool us into believing that technology somehow moves under its own power. Genetic technologies such as cloning do not evolve on their own. They only go where human beings decide to take them.

Part of the reason for despair in the face of the genetic genie is that humanity has done an abysmal job controlling the negative effects of other technological revolutions. Whether it is the depletion of the ozone, the ghastly effects of Chernobyl and Three Mile Island, the terror of the Cold War induced by the creation of atomic weapons, the presence of chemical and biological weapons in the hands of tinpot dictators, or the effects of the automobile on the air we breathe, to many humanity appears to be batting zero when it comes to reining in the downside of technology. It does not help to discover that the earliest experiments involving human embryo cloning at George Washington University in Washington, D.C., were conducted outside the standard regulations governing human experimentation or that the field of human reproductive technology remains nearly completely unregulated and unaccountable (see chapters 1 and 4) decades after the birth of the first test tube baby. Nor is it easy to put any faith in science's ability to control the impulse to clone when so many scientists had denied that such an achievement was even remotely possible in a mammal much less a primate. Some of the despair over the control of cloning issued directly from the fact that the public felt deceived by assurances that successful cloning was so far in the future that no one really had to worry.

The fear that technology is beyond our control becomes all the stronger when the society with the greatest ability to utilize the genetic revolution, the United States, seems the least able to reach moral consensus about how to do so and more likely than any other society on the globe to let the marketplace take the helm. If it is only the market that will tell the cloning genie what to do, then many Americans believe there is absolutely no chance that greed and self-interest will not lead directly to the irresponsible application of human cloning.

But the fact is, advances in biomedicine have been modulated by moral concerns. There are a number of technologies which have been shaped and controlled by law, regulation, and societal oversight.

Human experimentation is governed by rules that make it impossible to treat human beings the way they were treated by researchers forty and fifty years ago, regardless of the benefits in knowledge or new discoveries that might be gained by putting such protections aside (Grodin and Glantz, 1994; Caplan, 1997c). The same is true of animal research. As earlier discussions in this book make clear, technologies such as the artificial heart, fetal tissue transplants, and animal xenografting have been slowed or stopped by moral concerns. It is simply not true that morality has no power over the biomedical juggernaut. What is true is that societies are loathe to exercise that power for fear that constricting inquiry may come at a huge cost in terms of knowledge lost, commercial advantage sacrificed, and useful inventions forgone. But that is a political and policy tradeoff each citizen and each government must make.

A lack of faith that cloning can be kept on any length leash, much less a short one, is also a symptom of a different problem—ignorance. Many Americans have no understanding of genetics, heredity, or biology, much less technical issues such as cloning. When told that scientists have cloned a sheep or a monkey, they have very little idea of how such a thing might happen. This lack of knowledge of genetics provides a powerful source of fuel for those who argue that we can never control cloning. No one is likely to believe that anyone can control what only a few understand.

The lack of knowledge of biology, genetics, and cloning provides fodder for the view that cloning is a direct threat to human individuality. In a society as obsessed with freedom, autonomy, and personal choice as the United States, values that pervade many of the discussions of other biomedical advances in this book, cloning is a grave threat. To copy or duplicate human beings is to take away what is seen as most precious or value about them—their individuality.

Does cloning threaten individuality? Not really. Even a cloned organism is not perfectly identical with its fellow clone. Each organism may have the same set of genetic instructions, but clones made from adult cells will undergo a very different set of experiences and environments than did their genetic forbear. Similarly, twins and triplets can have the exact same genetic programming, but there is no doubt that development and environment turn them into different persons. For all the similarities that scientists find among twins, there are still obvious and important differences in their thoughts, emotions, personalities, and behavior. We are not our genes, and cloning genes is not the same as cloning our minds.

The copying metaphor used in describing cloning is often the copying of the Xerox machine. Cloning is much more akin to the copying of computer programs. Tens of millions of computers have copies of the same software programs. Still, despite these common programs, their outputs vary a great deal depending on what purpose they are used for and what input is fed into the software. Having a common biological program is no more a guarantee of a common output than having the same copy of a computer game is a guarantee that those who play it will get to the same outcome. Ignorance about the way genes govern bodies, behavior, and traits, in combination with a misunderstanding of how genes work and a powerful belief in genetic reductionism, drives anxiety about cloning very quickly to uncomfortable levels.

So, is there any reason to worry about cloning? Certainly there is. This is a technology that can and should be applied to animals. Turning away from all forms of cloning would be to step back from advances in animal breeding that could lead to the more efficient production of food and valuable biological materials as well as to useful ways to preserve endangered species. Cloning is a technology that probably should not be applied to people. In understanding why not, we need to have available the facts and moral values that make it repugnant to do to a human embryo what might be moral to do to a cow or sheep or condor embryo. Much of the difference in the morality of using cloning hinges on the fact that cloning bodies is of far more value for the production of milk, meat, and hides than it is for the production of children. And some of the moral difference hinges on the fact that copying goats or baboons will not saddle them with psychological and emotional baggage of the sort that will immediately confront human beings who grow up knowing they have been asexually created in the image of another person. There may be good reasons for creating human beings in this way, but it is very hard to imagine what they are. Until such time as someone can make a persuasive moral case, society should take the steps necessary to ensure that the burden of justifying human cloning falls upon those who seek to try.

ACKNOWLEDGMENTS

Some of the material in this book has appeared in somewhat different form in the following articles or essays.

"How Should Science Deal with Data from Unethical Research?" from *The Journal of NIH Research* May 1993: 5 (5) 22–26.

"Hard Cases Make Bad Law," in A. Caplan, R. Blank, and J. Merrick, eds., *Compelled Compassion* (Totowa, NJ: Humana Press, 1992).

"Will Assisted Suicide Kill Hospice?" in *Hospice Journal*, Volume 12:2, 1997.

"Odds and Ends: Trust and the Debate Over Medical Futility," in *Annals of Internal Medicine* October 15, 1996: 125 (8) 1202–04.

"Is Xenografting Morally Wrong?" in *Transplantation Proceedings*, 1992: 24 (2) 722–27.

Arthur L. Caplan (with C. Van Buren and N. Tilney), "Financial Compensation for Cadaver Organ Donation: Good Idea or Anathema?" in *Transplantation Proceedings* 1993: 25 (4) 2740–42.

"Am I My Brother's Keeper?" in *Suffolk University Law Review* December 1993: 27 (4) 1195–1208.

"The Ethics of Casting the First Stone: Personal Responsibility, Rationing and Transplants,"in *Alcoholism: Clinical and Experimental Research* 1994; 18 (2): 219–21. Published by Williams & Wilkins. With permission.

"The Ethical Implications of the Corporatization of American Health Care," in Ellen D. Baer, Claire M. Fagin, and Suzanne Gordon, eds. *The Abandonment of the Patient* (New York: Springer Publishing Co., 1997).

Adapted from Arthur Caplan's "Concepts of Health, Illness, and Disease," in Veatch: *Medical Ethics* © 1997 Boston: Jones and Bartlett Publishers. With permission.

"Can Philosophy Cure What Ails the Medical Model?" in Robert L. Berg and Joseph S. Cassells, eds., *The Second Fifty Years: Promoting Health and Preventing Disability* (Washington, DC: National Academy of Sciences Presses, 1990).

"If Gene Therapy Is the Cure, What Is the Disease?" in George J. Annas and Sherman Elias, eds., *Gene Mapping: Using Law and Ethics as Guides*. Used by permission of Oxford University Press.

REFERENCES AND
SUGGESTED READINGS

Abadi, R., and E. Pascal. 1989. "The Recognition and Management of Albinism." *Ophthalmology and Physiological Optometry* 9: 3–15.

Adams, D. P. 1991. *The Greatest Good to the Greatest Number: Penicillin Rationing on the American Home Front, 1940–1945.* New York: Peter Lang.

Adams, M. B. 1990. *The Wellborn Science: Eugenics in Germany, France, Brazil and Russia.* New York: Oxford University Press.

Advisory Committee on Human Radiation Experiments. *Final Report.* Washington, D.C., October 1995.

Anderson, W. F. 1989. "Human Gene Therapy: Why Draw a Line?" *Journal of Medicine and Philosophy* 14: 681–93.

Andrusko, D. 1991. *NRL News.*

Angell, M. 1992. "Editorial Responsibility: Protecting Human Rights by Restricting Publication of Unethical Research." In Annas and Grodin, 276–85.

Annas, G. J. 1985. "The Prostitute, the Playboy and the Poet: Rationing Schemes for Organ Transplantation." *American Journal of Public Health* 75: 187–89.

Annas, G. J. 1993. *Standard of Care: The Law of American Bioethics.*

Annas, G. J., A. L. Caplan, and S. Elias. 1996. "The Politics of Human Embryo Research." *New England Journal of Medicine* 334, 20: 1329–32.

Annas, G. J., and M. A. Grodin, eds. 1992. *The Nazi Doctors and the Nuremberg Code.* New York: Oxford University Press.

Anonymous. 1995. "AMA Reinstates Restrictive Infant Donor Policy." *Lancet,* December 16, 1618.

Anspach, R. R. 1993. *Deciding Who Lives.* Berkeley: University of California Press.

Arnold, R. M., and S. J. Youngner. 1993. "Back to the Future: Obtaining Organs from Non-heart-beating Cadavers." *Kennedy Institute of Ethics Journal* 3, 3: 103–12.

Asch, D. 1996. "The Role of Critical Care Nurses in Euthanasia and Assisted Suicide." *New England Journal of Medicine* 334, 20: 1374–79.

Asch, D., and M. Fine, eds. 1988. "Moving Disability beyond Stigma." *Journal of Social Issues* 44, 1.

Atterbury, C. E. 1986. "The Alcoholic in the Lifeboat: Should Drinkers Be Candidates for Liver Transplantation?" *Journal of Clinical Gastroenterology* 8: 1–4.

Baer, E. D., C. Fagin, and S. Gordon, eds. 1996. *Abandonment of the Patient.* New York: Springer.

Baer, E. D., and S. Gordon. 1994. "Money Managers Are Unraveling the Tapestry of Nursing." *American Journal of Nursing* 94, 10: 38–40.

Baker, L. A. 1995. "Bargaining for Public Assistance." *Denver University Law Review* 72: 949–62.

Baum, B., D. Bernstein, V. A. Starnes, P. Oyer, P. Pitlick, E. Stinson, and N. Shumway. 1991. "Pediatric Heart Transplantation at Stanford: Results of a 15-year Experience." *Pediatrics* 88, 2: 203–14.

Bay, B., and M. Burgess. 1991. "A Survey of Calgary Paediatricians' Attitudes regarding the Treatment of Defective Newborns." *Bioethics* 5, 2 (April): 139–49.

Bayer, R. 1981. *Homosexuality and American Psychiatry.* New York: Basic.

Bernstein, B. 1984. "The Misguided Quest for the Artificial Heart." *Technology Review* 87: 13–17.

Blakeslee, S., ed. 1986. *Human Heart Replacement: A New Challenge for Physicians and Reporters.* Washington, D.C., Foundation for American Communications.

Blank, R. 1988. *Rationing Medicine.* New York: Columbia University Press.

Bleich, J. D. 1993. "Survey of Recent Halakhic Periodical Literature: Compelling Tissue Donations." *Tradition* 27, 3: 59–89.

Blendon, R. J., et al. 1992. "Should Physicians Aid Their Patients in Dying?" *Journal of the American Medical Association* 267, May 20: 2658–81.

Bonet, H., R. Manez, D. Kramer, H. I. Wright, J. S. Gavaler, N. Baddour, and D. H. Van Thiel. 1993. "Liver Transplantation for Alcoholic Liver Disease: Survival of Patients Transplanted with Alcoholic Hepatitis plus Cirrhosis as Compared to Those with Cirrhosis Alone." *Alcoholism* 18, 2: 147–53.

Boone, S. S. 1992. "Slavery and Contract Motherhood: A Radicalized Objection to Autonomy Arguments." In H. B. Holmes, ed., *Issues in Reproductive Technology.* New York: Garland, 349–66.

Boorse, C. 1975. "On the Distinction between Disease and Illness." *Philosophy and Public Affairs* 5: 49–68.

Boorse, C. 1976. "What a Theory of Mental Health Should Be." *Philosophy of Science* 44: 542–73.

Boorse, C. 1987. "Concepts of Health." In D. Van De Veer and T. Regan, eds., *Health Care Ethics.* Philadelphia: Temple University Press, 359–94.

Bopp, J., and J. T. Burtchaell. 1988. "Human Fetal Tissue Transplantation Research Panel: Statement of Dissent." In *Report of the Human Fetal Tissue Transplantation Research Panel,* vol. 1. Bethesda, Md.: National Institutes of Health.

Brahams, D., and M. Brahams. 1983. "The Arthur Case: A Proposal for Legislation." *Journal of Medical Ethics* 9: 12–17.

Brandt, A. M. 1978. "Racism and Research: The Case of the Tuskegee Syphilis Study." *Hastings Center Report* 8, 6: 21–29.

Brinster, R. 1995. "Spermatogenesis following Male Germ Cell Transplantation." *Proceedings of the National Academy of Sciences* 91, 24: 11298–312.

Buckingham, R. W. 1996. *The Handbook of Hospice Care.* Amherst, N.Y.: Prometheus.

Buttle, N. 1991. "Prostitutes, Workers and Kidneys." *Journal of Medical Ethics* 17: 97–98.

Callahan, D. 1993. *The Troubled Dream of Life.* New York: Simon and Schuster.

Callahan, D. 1995. "Terminating Life-Sustaining Treatment of the Demented." *Hastings Center Report* 25, 6: 25–31.

Callender, C. O. 1987. "Organ Donation in the Black Population: Where Do We Go from Here?" *Transplantation Proceedings* 19: 36–40.

Caplan, A. L. 1983. "Organ Transplants: The Costs of Success." *Hastings Center Report* 13: 23–32.

Caplan, A. L. 1984a. "Is It a Life?" *The Nation* 238, 2 (January 21): 37.

Caplan, A. L. 1984b. "Organ Procurement: It's Not in the Cards." *Hastings Center Report* 14, 5: 6–9.

Caplan, A. L. 1985. "Ethical Issues Raised by Research involving Xenografts." *Journal of the American Medical Association* 254, 23: 3339–43.

Caplan, A. L. 1987a. "Imperiled Newborns." *Hastings Center Report* 17: 6, 15–32.

Caplan, A. L. 1987b. "Should Fetuses or Infants Be Used as Organ Donors?" *Bioethics* 1, 2: 119–40.

Caplan, A. L. 1988. "Professional Arrogance and Public Misunderstanding." *Hastings Center Report* 18, 2: 34–37.

Caplan, A. L. 1989a. "The Concepts of Health and Disease." In R. Veatch, ed., *Medical Ethics.* Boston: Jones and Bartlett, 49–63.

Caplan, A. L. 1989b. "Fragile Trust: The Success and Failure of Required Request Laws and the Procurement of Organs and Tissues from Children and Adults." In H. Kaufman, ed., *Pediatric Brain Death and Organ Procurement.* New York: Plenum, 299–307.

Caplan, A. L. 1989c. "Problems in the Policies and Criteria Used to Allocate Organs for Transplantation in the United States." *Transplantation Proceedings* 21, 3: 3381–87.

Caplan, A. L. 1989d. "Sin, Virtue and Renal Failure." *American Kidney Fund Newsletter* 6: 3.

Caplan, A. L. 1990. "Organ Donation Should Be Considered a Moral Obligation." *Physicians Weekly* 7: 1.

Caplan, A. L. 1991. "Assume Nothing: The Current State of Cadaver Organ and Tissue Donation in the United States." *Journal of Transplant Coordination* 1, 2: 78–83.

Caplan, A. L. 1992a. *If I Were a Rich Man Could I Buy a Pancreas?* Bloomington: Indiana University Press.

Caplan, A. L. 1992b. "When Evil Intrudes." *Hastings Center Report* 22, 6: 29–32.

Caplan, A. L., ed. 1992c. *When Medicine Went Mad: Bioethics and the Holocaust.* Totowa, N.J.: Humana.

Caplan, A. L. 1993. "The Concepts of Health, Illness and Disease." In W. F. Bynum and R. Porter, eds., *Encyclopaedia of the History of Medicine.* London: Routledge, 233–48.

Caplan, A. L. 1995a. *Moral Matters: Ethical Issues in Medicine and Science.* New York: Wiley.

Caplan, A. L. 1995b. "Straight Talk about Rationing." *Annals of Internal Medicine* 122, 10: 795–96.

Caplan, A. L. 1996a. "Allwood Eight." *St. Paul Pioneer Press,* August 10, p. 12.

Caplan, A. L. 1996b. "Odds, Ends and Trust." *Annals of Internal Medicine* 125, 8: 1202–4.

Caplan, A. L. 1996c. "Why Is It So Hard to Be Dead in America?" *Philadelphia Inquirer,* September 6, p. 14.

Caplan, A. L. 1996d. "Why Is Kevorkian an American Hero?" *Philadelphia Inquirer,* March 17, p. 12.

Caplan, A. L. 1997a. "The Ethical Implications of the Corporatization of American Health Care." In C. Fagin, ed., *The Abandonment of the Patient.* New York: Springer, 87–101.

Caplan, A. L. 1997b. "The Ethics of Gatekeeping in Rehabilitation Medicine." *Journal of Head Rehabilitation Trauma* 12, 1, 29–37.

Caplan, A. L. 1997. "Cloning and the Biotech Century." *Business Week Online.* Transcript of March 2 online conference.

Caplan, A. L., and R. Bayer. 1985. *Ethical, Legal and Policy Issues Pertaining to Solid Organ Procurement.* New York: Empire Blue Cross/Blue Shield.

Caplan, A. L., H. T. Engelhardt, and J. McCartney, eds. 1981. *The Concepts of Health and Disease.* Reading, Mass.: Addison-Wesley.

Caplan, A. L., L. Siminoff, B. Arnold, and B. Virnig. 1992. "Increasing Organ and Tissue Donation: What Are Our Options, What Are the Obstacles?" Paper presented at Surgeon General's Workshop on Organ Donation. Washington, D.C.

Caplan, A. L., C. Van Buren, and N. L. Tilney. 1993. "Financial Compensation for Cadaver Organ Donation." *Transplantation Proceedings* 25, 4: 2740–42.

Caplan, A. L., and B. Virnig. 1990. "Is Altruism Enough?" *Critical Care Clinics* 6, 4: 1007–18.

Caplan, A. L., and P. Welvang. 1989. "Are Required Request Laws Working?" *Clinical Transplantation* 3, 3: 170–76.

Carey, J. 1997. "The Biotech Century." *Business Week,* March 10, 72–76.

Carson, E. 1996. "Paying Organ Donors Would Increase Availability." *Philadelphia Inquirer,* December 27, p. 12.

Cassel, C. K., and D. E. Meier. 1990. "Morals and Moralism in the Debate over Euthanasia and Assisted Suicide." *New England Journal of Medicine,* September 13, 750–51.

Chan, C. K. 1987. "Eugenics on the Rise: A Report from Singapore." In R. Chadwick, ed., *Ethics, Reproduction and Genetic Control.* London: Routledge, 164–72.

Charo, R. A. 1995. "The Hunting of the Snark: The Moral Status of Embryos,

Right-to-Lifers and Third World Women." *Stanford Law and Policy Review* 6: 11–38.

Charo, R. A., and D. Wikler. 1994. Letter to the Editor. *New York Times,* January 14, p. 14.

Childress, J. 1982. *Who Should Decide?* New York: Oxford University Press.

Christakis, N. A., and D. A. Asch. 1993. "Biases in How Physicians Choose to Withdraw Life Support." *Lancet* 342: 642–46.

Christensen, K., S. Kelleher, M. Nicolosi, and D. Parrish. 1995. "Doctors Raise Doubts about Regulation." *Orange County Register,* November 22, p. 1.

Clouser, K., C. Culver, and B. Gert. 1981. "Malady: A New Treatment of Disease." *Hastings Center Report* 11, 3: 29–37.

Cohen, B. 1994. Introduction. *Eurotransplant Newsletter* 113 (February): 1.

Cohen, C., and M. Benjamin. 1991. "Alcoholics and Liver Transplantation." *Journal of the American Medical Association* 265: 1299–1301.

Cohen, L. R. 1989. "Increasing the Supply of Transplant Organs: The Virtues of a Futures Market." *George Washington Law Review* 58, 1–51.

Cohen, L. R. 1996. "Markets and the Blood Supply." In Institute of Medicine, *Blood Donors and the Supply of Blood,* 41–45. Washington, D.C.: NAS Press.

Collins, J. A. 1994. "Reproductive Technology: The Price of Progress." *New England Journal of Medicine* 331: 270–71.

Conference of European Health Ministers. 1987. "Removal of Organs from Living Donors." Final Communique, appendix II, Paris, November 17.

Connors, R. B., and M. L. Smith. 1996. "Religious Insistence on Medical Treatment: Christian Theology and Re-imagination." *Hastings Center Report* 26, 4: 23–30.

Consultants to the Advisory Committee to the Director. 1988. *Report of the Human Fetal Tissue Transplantation Research Panel,* vol. 1. Bethesda, Md.: National Institutes of Health.

Council of Europe. 1996. Convention on Human Rights and Biomedicine.

Council of the Transplantation Society. 1985. "Commercialisation in Transplantation: The Problems and Some Guidelines for Practice." *Lancet,* September, 715–16.

Covington, S. 1995. "The Role of the Mental Health Professional in Reproductive Medicine." *Fertility and Sterility* 64: 895–97.

Craig, O. 1996. "Couple Wants Their Dead Daughter to Be a Mother." *London Times,* December 29, 10–12.

Crocker, A., and M. Cullinane. 1972. "Families under Stress." *Postgraduate Medicine,* March, 223–29.

Culver, C. M., and B. Gert. 1982. *Philosophy in Medicine.* New York: Oxford University Press.

Davis, D. S. 1995. "Embryos Created for Research Purposes." *Kennedy Institute of Ethics Journal* 5, 4: 343–55.

Davis, J. 1991. "94 Percent Awareness and Still Not Enough Donors." Paper presented at Surgeon General's Workshop on Increasing Organ Donation. Washington, D.C., July 8.

Dellinger, A. M., and P. C. Kuszler. 1995. "Infants: Public Policy and Legal Issues." In *Encyclopedia of Bioethics,* rev. ed. New York: Macmillan, 1214–21.

Department of Health and Human Services. 1983. "Nondiscrimination on the Basis of Handicap." *Federal Register* 48: 9630–32.

Department of Health and Human Services. 1985. "Child Abuse and Neglect Prevention and Treatment Program and Services and Treatment for Disabled Infants: Model Guidelines for Health Care Providers to Establish Infant Care Review Committees." *Federal Register* 50: 14878–901.

DeVries, W., et al. 1984. "Clinical Use of the Total Artificial Heart." *New England Journal of Medicine* 310: 273–78.

Donaldson, T. 1993. "Morally Privileged Relationships." In D. T. Meyers, K. Kipnis, and C. F. Murphy, Jr., eds., *Kindred Matters*. Ithaca: Cornell University Press, 21–41.

Duff, R., and A. Campbell. 1973. "Moral and Ethical Dilemmas in the Special-Care Nursery." *New England Journal of Medicine* 289: 890–94.

Duster, T. 1990. *Backdoor to Eugenics*. New York: Routledge.

Edwards, B. C. 1991. "Evaluating Required Request: Lessons to Date." *Journal of Transplant Coordination* 1, 2: 84–90.

Elias, S., and G. J. Annas. 1987. *Reproductive Genetics and the Law*. New York: Yearbook Medical.

Elick, B. A., D. E. R. Sutherland, K. Gillingham, and J. S. Najarian. 1990. "Use of Distant Relatives and Living Unrelated Donors: A Strategy to Increase the Application of Kidney Transplantation to Treat Chronic Renal Failure." *Transplantation Proceedings* 22, 2: 343–44.

Elliott, D., and F. Endt. 1995. "Twins with Two Fathers." *Newsweek,* July 3, p. 38.

Emanuel, L. L. 1995. "Reexamining Death: The Asymptotic Model and a Bounded Zone Definition." *Hastings Center Report* 25, 4: 27–35.

Engelhardt, H. T. 1986. *The Foundations of Bioethics*. New York: Oxford University Press.

Engelhardt, H. T., and A. L. Caplan, eds. 1987. *Scientific Controversies*. New York: Cambridge University Press.

Eurotransplant Foundation. 1991. "Statistics." *Eurotransplant Newsletter* 87, 7: 1–2.

Evans, M. 1989. "Organ Donations Should Not Be Restricted to Relatives." *Journal of Medical Ethics* 15: 17–20.

Evans, R. W., and D. L. Manninen. 1988. "U.S. Public Opinion concerning the Procurement and Distribution of Donor Organs." *Transplantation Proceedings* 20, 3, 781–85.

Faber-Langendoen, K. 1991. "Resuscitation of the Patient with Metastatic Cancer: Is Transient Benefit Still Futile?" *Archives of Internal Medicine* 151: 235–39.

Faber-Langendoen, K., A. L. Caplan, and P. B. McGlave. 1993. "Survival of Adult Bone Marrow Transplant Patients Receiving Mechanical Ventilation: A Case for Restricted Use." *Bone Marrow Transplant* 12: 501–7.

Fabrega, H. 1972. "Concepts of Disease: Logical Features and Social Implications." *Perspectives in Biology and Medicine* 5: 538–617.

Faden, R. R., and T. L. Beauchamp. 1986. *A History and Theory of Informed Consent*. New York: Oxford University Press.

Fingarette, H. 1988. *Heavy Drinking: The Myth of Alcoholism as a Disease.* Berkeley: University of California Press.

Flew, A. 1983. "Mental Health, Mental Disease, Mental Illness: The Medical Model." In P. Bean, ed., *Mental Illness.* New York: Wiley.

Food and Drug Administration. 1996. Fact Sheet on Xenotransplantation. Rockville, Md., September 20.

Foucault, M. 1965. *Madness and Civilization.* London: Tavistock.

Fox, R. C., and J. P. Swazey. 1992. *Spare Parts.* New York: Oxford University Press.

Freyer, F. J. 1995. "Women and Infants Face Third Suit on Missing Embryos." *Providence Journal-Bulletin,* November 1, p. 1B.

Freudenheim, M. 1996. "As Insurers Cut Fees, Doctors Shift to Elective Procedures." *New York Times,* August 24, pp. 1, 12.

Frohock, F. M. 1986. *Special Care.* Chicago: University of Chicago Press.

Gamble, V. N. 1991. "Race, Gender and Class in American Medicine." Speech at the symposium Race, Prejudice and Health Care: The Legacy of the Tuskegee Study, Minneapolis, June 1.

Garry, D., A. L. Caplan, D. E. Vawter, and W. Kearney. 1992. "Are There Really Alternatives to the Use of Fetal Tissue from Elective Abortions in Transplantation Research?" *New England Journal of Medicine* 327, 22: 1592–96.

Gaul, Gilbert. 1989. "The Artificial Heart Juggernaut." *Hastings Center Report* 19: 24–31.

Gerry, M. 1985. "The Civil Rights of Handicapped Infants." *Issues in Law and Medicine* 1: 15–66.

Gerson, F. 1987. "Refining the Law of Organ Donation: Lessons from the French Law of Presumed Consent." *NYU Journal of International Law and Policy* 19: 1013–27.

Gervais, K. G. 1986. *Redefining Death.* New Haven: Yale University Press.

Goosens, W. 1980. "Values, Health and Medicine." *Philosophy of Science* 47: 133–54.

Gosden, R. G., D. T. Baird, J. C. Wade, and R. Webb. 1994. "Restoration of Fertility to Oophorectomized Sheep by Ovarian Autografts Stored at -196 C." *Human Reproduction* 9: 597–603.

Grodin, M. A., and L. H. Glantz, eds. 1994. *Children as Research Subjects.* New York: Oxford University Press.

Guillemin, J., and L. Holmstrom. 1987. *Mixed Blessings.* New York: Oxford University Press.

Haas, J., A. L. Caplan, and D. Callahan. 1987. "Ethical and Policy Issues in Rehabilitation Medicine." *Hastings Center Report* 17: 1–20.

Halevy, A., and B. A. Brody. 1993. "Brain Death: Reconciling Definitions." *Annals of Internal Medicine* 119: 519–25.

Halevy, A., and B. A. Brody. 1996. "A Multi-institution Collaborative Policy on Medical Futility." *Journal of the American Medical Association* 276: 571–74.

Hall, S. S. 1990. "James Watson and the Search for Biology's 'Holy Grail.'" *Smithsonian.*

Haller, M. H. 1963. *Eugenics: Hereditarian Attitudes in American Thought*. New Brunswick, N.J.: Rutgers University Press.

Hamburger, J., and J. Crosnier. 1968: "Moral and Ethical Problems in Transplantation." In F. Rapaport, T. Felix, and J. Dausset, eds., *Human Transplantation*. New York: Grune & Stratton, 37–44.

Hansmann, H. 1989. "The Economics and Ethics of Markets for Human Organs." *Journal of Health Politics, Policy and Law*, 57–71.

Harding, S., ed. 1993. *The "Racial" Economy of Science*. Bloomington: Indiana University Press.

Hart v. Brown, 29 Conn.Supp. 368; 289 A. 2d 386, 1972.

Harvey, J. 1990. "Paying Organ Donors." *Journal of Medical Ethics* 16: 117–19.

Herrnstein, R. J., and C. Murray. 1994. *The Bell Curve: Intelligence and Class Structure in American Life*. New York: Free Press.

Hessing, D. J., and H. Elffers. 1987. "Attitude toward Death, Fear of Being Declared Dead Too Soon and Donation of Organs after Death." *Omega* 17: 115–26.

Hoffmeister, B., B. Freedman, and G. Fraser, eds. 1989. *Clinical Ethics: Theory and Practice*. Clifton, N.J.: Humana.

In re Richardson, 284 So. 2d 185 (La Ct App.), cert denied, 284 So. 2d 338 (La. 1973).

Institute of Medicine. 1991. *The Artificial Heart: Prototypes, Policies and Patients*. Washington, D.C.: National Academy Press.

Institute of Medicine. 1996. *Xenotransplantation: Science, Ethics and Public Policy*. Washington, D.C.: National Academy Press.

Jasper, J. M., and D. Nelkin. 1992. *The Animal Rights Crusade*. New York: Free Press.

Jennings, B. 1995. "Individual Rights and the Human Good in Hospice." *Hastings Center Report* 25, 1: 6–8.

John Paul II. 1991. "Statement on Organ Transplantation." International Congress of the Society for Organ Sharing, Rome, June 20.

Johny, K. V., J. Nesim, N. Namboori, and R. K. Gupta. 1990. "Values Gained and Lost in Live Unrelated Renal Transplantation." *Transplantation Proceedings* 22, 3: 915–17.

Jones, J. H. 1981. *Bad Blood: The Tuskegee Syphilis Experiment*. New York: Free Press.

Kahn, Patricia. 1993. "A Grisly Archive of Key Cancer Data." *Science*, January 22, 448–51.

Kandela, P. 1991. "India: Kidney Bazaar." *Lancet* 337: 1534.

Kass, L. 1975. "Regarding the End of Medicine and the Pursuit of Health." *Public Interest* 40: 11–42.

Kendall, P. 1997. "Human Cloning Debate: Why Do It? Who'd Be Hurt? Should It Be Legal?" *Chicago Tribune*, February 23, 8–9.

Kendell, R. 1975. "The Concept of Disease and Its Implications for Psychiatry." *British Journal of Psychiatry* 127: 305–15.

Kevles, D. 1985. *In the Name of Eugenics*. New York: Knopf.

Kevorkian, J. 1992. "A Controlled Auction Market Is a Practical Solution to the Shortage of Transplantable Organs." *Medicine and Law* 11 (1–2): 47–55.

King, L. 1984. *Medical Thinking*. Princeton: Princeton University Press.

King, W. 1995. "Law Can't Stop Abuse, Infertility Doctors Say." *Seattle Times,* October 10, p. B1.

Klass, P. 1989. "The Perfect Baby?" *New York Times Magazine,* January 29.

Kokkedee, W. 1992. "Kidney Procurement Policies in the Eurotransplant Region." *Social Science and Medicine* 35, 2: 177–82.

Kolata, G. 1994. "Fetal Ovary Transplant Is Envisioned." *New York Times,* January 6.

Kolata, G. 1995. "Transplants, Morality and Mickey." *New York Times,* June 11, p. 5.

Kolker, A., and B. M. Burke. 1994. *Prenatal Testing: A Sociological Perspective.* Westport, Conn.: Bergin and Garvey.

Koop, C. E. 1991. Personal communication.

Koppelman, L., T. Irons, and A. Koppelman. 1988. "Neonatologists Judge the 'Baby Doe' Regulations." *New England Journal of Medicine* 318: 677–83.

Kreis, H. 1985. "Why Living Related Donors Should Not Be Used Whenever Possible." *Transplantation Proceedings* 17: 1510–14.

Krimsky, S., and R. Hubbard. 1995. "The Business of Research." *Hastings Center Report* 25, 1: 41–43.

Levenson, J. L., and M. E. Olbrish. 1993. "Psychosocial Evaluation of Organ Transplant Candidates." *Psychosomatics* 34: 314–23.

Levine, R. 1986. *Human Experimentation.* 2d ed. Baltimore: Urban and Schwartzenberg.

Lindee, M. S. 1994. *Suffering Made Real: American Science and the Survivors at Hiroshima.* Chicago: University of Chicago Press.

Little v. Little, 576 S.W. 2d 493 (Texas, 1979).

Lorber, J. 1972. "Spina Bifida Cystica—Results of Treatment of 270 Consecutive Cases with Criteria for Selection for the Future." *Archives of Diseases of Children* 47: 854–73.

Lowance, D. L. 1993. "Factors and Guidelines to Be Considered in Offering Treatment to Patients with End-stage Renal Disease: A Personal Opinion." *American Journal of Kidney Diseases* 21, 6: 679–83.

Lucey, M. R. 1993. "Liver Transplantation for the Alcoholic Patient." *Gastroenterology Clinics of North America* 22: 243–56.

Lucey, M. R., and T. P. Beresford. 1992. "Alcoholic Liver Disease: To Transplant or Not to Transplant?" *Alcohol and Alcoholism* 27: 103–108.

Majeske, R. A., L. S. Parker, and J. E. Frader. 1996. "In Search of an Ethical Framework for Consideration of Decisions regarding Live Donation." In B. Spielman, ed., *Organ and Tissue Donation.* Carbondale: Southern Illinois University Press, 90–101.

Manga, P. 1986. "Waiting Impatiently in the Queue: Should We Have a Commercial Market for Organs?" University of Ottawa Working Paper 86–25.

Manitoba Law Reform Commission. 1986. Report on the Human Tissue Act. Winnipeg.

Manning, W. G., E. B. Keeler, J. P. Newhouse, E. M. Sloss, and J. Wasserman. 1991. *The Costs of Poor Health Habits.* Cambridge: Harvard University Press.

Margolis, J. 1976. "The Concept of Disease." *Journal of Medicine and Philosophy* 1: 238–55.

Marshall, P. A., D. C. Thomasma, and A. S. Daar. 1996. "Marketing Human Organs: The Autonomy Paradox." *Theoretical Medicine* 17, 1: 1–18.

Martyn, S., R. Wright, and L. Clark. 1988. "Required Request for Organ Donation: Moral, Clinical and Legal Problems." *Hastings Center Report* 18, 2: 27–33.

Matas, A. J., J. Arras, J. Muyskens, V. Tellis, and F. J. Veith. 1985. "A Proposal for Cadaver Organ Procurement: Routine Removal with Right of Informed Refusal." *Journal of Health Politics, Policy and Law* 10, 2: 231–44.

Maugh, T. H. 1997. "Oregon Scientists Report Cloning Monkeys; Research Success with Embryos Suggests Process May Be Readily Transferable to Humans." *Los Angeles Times,* March 2, 27.

May, W. F. 1988. "Religious Obstacles and Warrants for the Donation of Body Parts." *Transplantation Proceedings* 20, 1: 1078–83.

McCormick, R. A. 1978. "Organ Transplantation: Ethical Principles." *Encyclopedia of Bioethics,* vol. 3., 1169–72.

McGee, G. 1997. *The Perfect Baby.* Lanham, Md.: Rowman and Littlefield.

Mechanic, D. 1996. "Trust and Managed Care." *Journal of the American Medical Association.*

Mechanic, D., and M. Schlesinger. 1996. "The Impact of Managed Care on Patients' Trust in Medical Care and Their Physicians." *Journal of the American Medical Association* 275: 1693–97.

Menzel, P. T. 1990. *Strong Medicine: The Ethical Rationing of Health Care.* New York: Oxford University Press.

Misbin, R. E., B. Jennings, D. Orentlicher, and M. Dewar, eds. 1995. *Health Care Crisis?* Frederick, Md.: University Publishing Group.

Moore v. Regents of the University of California, 271 Cal. Rptr. 146, 1990.

Moreno, J. D. 1995. *Deciding Together.* New York: Oxford University Press.

Moss, A. H., and M. Siegler. 1991. "Should Alcoholics Compete Equally for Liver Transplants? *Journal of the American Medical Association* 265: 1295–98.

Muller-Hill, B. 1988. *Murderous Science.* Oxford: Oxford University Press.

Murphy, E. A. 1976. *The Logic of Medicine.* Baltimore: Johns Hopkins University Press.

Murphy, T. F., and M. A. Lappe, eds. 1994. *Justice and the Human Genome Project.* Berkeley: University of California Press.

Murray, T., and A. L. Caplan, eds. 1985. *Which Babies Shall Live?* Clifton, N.J.: Humana.

Mydans, S. 1995. "Fertility Clinic Told to Close Amid Complaints." *New York Times,* May 29, p. 7.

National Heart and Lung Institute. 1973. *The Totally Implantable Artificial Heart: Economic, Ethical, Legal, Medical, Psychiatric, and Social Implications.* Washington, D.C.: Department of Health, Education, and Welfare.

National Kidney Foundation. 1991. "Controversies in Organ Donation: Financial Incentives." Consensus Conference, New Orleans, February 25–26.

National Organ Transplant Act, 1984. Pub L. No. 98–507, 3USC *301.

New Scientist. 1991. "Pioneer Killed." July 13, p. 19.

Nimz, M. 1989. "How Protected Are Infants with Disabilities?" In D. Andrusko, ed., *The Triumph of Hope.* Washington, D.C.: National Right to Life, 145–57.

Nuffield Council on Bioethics. 1996. *Animal to Human Transplants*. London: Nuffield Council on Bioethics.

Office of Technology Assessment. 1994. "Identifying Health Technologies That Work: Searching for Evidence." OTA-H-608. Washington, D.C.: Government Printing Office.

Orentlicher, D. 1996. "Psychosocial Assessment of Organ Transplant Candidates and the Americans with Disabilities Act. *General Hospital Psychiatry* 18, 5–12.

Overall, C. 1987. *Ethics and Human Reproduction*. New York: Routledge, Chapman and Hall.

Pechura, C. M., and D. P. Rall, eds. 1993. *Veterans at Risk: The Health Effects of Mustard Gas and Lewisite*. Washington D.C.: National Academy Press.

Pellegrino, E. D., and D. C. Thomasma. 1988. *For the Patient's Good*. Oxford: Oxford University Press.

Peters, T. G. 1991a. "Life or Death: The Issue of Payment in Cadaveric Organ Donation." *Journal of the American Medical Association* 265: 1302–5.

Peters, T. G. 1991b. "Should Cash Payments Be Made to Organ Donors' Next of Kin—Yes." *Physician's Weekly* 8, 14 (April 15): 1.

Post, S. G. 1995. "Baby K: Medical Futility and the Free Exercise of Religion." *Journal of Law and Medical Ethics* 23: 20–26.

Powell, T., and A. Hecimovic. 1985. "Baby Doe and the Search for a Quality of Life." *Exceptional Children*, January, 15–23.

President's Commission for the Study of Ethical Problems in Medicine and Biomedical and Behavioral Research. 1982. *Making Health Care Decisions*, vol. 1. Washington, D.C.: Government Printing Office.

Proctor, R. 1988. *Racial Hygiene*. Cambridge, Mass.: Harvard University Press.

Pross, C. 1992. "Nazi Doctors, German Medicine and Historical Truth." In G. J. Annas and M. A. Grodin, eds., *The Nazi Doctors and the Nuremberg Code*. New York: Oxford University Press, 32–52.

Quill, T. 1993. *Death and Dignity*. New York: Norton.

Raia, S., J. R. Nery, and S. Mies. 1989. "Liver Transplantation from Live Donors." *Lancet*, August 26, 497.

Ramsey, P. 1970. *The Patient as Person*. New Haven: Yale University Press.

Rapaport, F. 1986. "The Case for a Living Emotionally Related International Kidney Donor Exchange Registry." *Transplantation Proceedings* 18: 5–9.

Rapp, R. 1988. "Moral Pioneers: Women, Men and Fetuses on a Frontier of Reproductive Technology." *Women and Health* 13, 1: 101–16.

Raymond, J. G. 1993. *Women As Wombs*. New York: Harper.

Regan, T., and P. Singer, eds. 1976. *Animal Rights and Human Obligations*. Englewood Cliffs, N.J.: Prentice-Hall.

Regan, T., and D. VanDeVeer, eds. 1982. *And Justice for All*. Totowa, N.J.: Rowman and Littlefield, 1982.

Reilly, P. R. 1991. *The Surgical Solution: A History of Involuntary Sterilization in the United States*. Baltimore: Johns Hopkins University Press.

Reznek, Lawrie. 1987. *The Nature of Disease*. London: Routledge and Kegan Paul.

Rhoden, N. 1986. "Treating Baby Doe: The Ethics of Uncertainty." *Hastings Center Report* 16: 34–42.

Rhoden, N., and J. Arras. 1985. "Withholding Treatment from Baby Doe: From

Discrimination to Child Abuse." *Milbank Memorial Fund Quarterly* 63: 18–51.

Rifkin, J. 1985a. *Declaration of a Heretic.* Boston: Routledge and Kegan Paul.

Rifkin, J. 1985b. "Perils of Genetic Engineering." *Resurgence* 109 (March-April): 4–7.

Robertson, J. A. 1995. "The Case of the Switched Embryos." *Hastings Center Report* 25, 6: 13–19.

Robertson, J. A. 1994. *Children of Choice.* Princeton: Princeton University Press.

Rosner, D. 1982. *A Once Charitable Enterprise: Hospitals and Health Care in Brooklyn and New York, 1885–1915.* New York: Cambridge University Press.

Rubenfeld, G. D., and S. W. Crawford. 1996. "Withdrawing Life Support in Mechanically Ventilated Bone Marrow Transplant Patients: A Case for Evidence Based Guidelines." *Annals of Internal Medicine* 125, 8: 625–33.

Sale, K. 1997. "Ban Cloning? Not a Chance." *New York Times,* March 7, A35.

Samet, J. M., D. M. Kutvirt, R. J. Waxweiler, and C. R. Key. 1984. "Uranium Mining and Lung Cancer in Navajo Men." *New England Journal of Medicine* 310, 23 (June 7): 1481–84.

Savitt, T. L. 1982. "The Use of Blacks for Medical Experimentation and Demonstration in the Old South." *Journal of Southern History* 48, 3: 331–48.

Scadding, J. 1967. "Diagnosis, the Clinician and the Computer." *Lancet* 2: 877–82.

Scadding, J. 1996. "Essentialism and Nominalism in Medicine." *Lancet* 348: 594–96.

Schmickle, S. 1997. "Cloning Debate Full of Mystery and Wonder." *Minneapolis Star and Tribune,* March 2, 1A.

Schneiderman, L. J., and N. S. Jecker. 1995. *Wrong Medicine: Doctors, Patients and Futile Treatment.* Baltimore: Johns Hopkins University Press.

Schneiderman, L. J., N. S. Jecker, and A. R. Jonsen. 1990. "Medical Futility: Its Meaning and Ethical Implications." *Annals of Internal Medicine* 112: 949–54.

Schneiderman, L. J., N. S. Jecker, and A. R. Jonsen. 1996. "Medical Futility: Response to Critiques." *Annals of Internal Medicine* 125, 8: 669–74.

Sedgwick, P. 1973. "Illness—Mental and Otherwise." *Hastings Center Studies* 1: 19–40.

Seelye, K. Q. 1997. "GOP Lawmaker Proposes Bill to Ban Human Cloning." *New York Times,* March 6, B12.

Sells, R. A., and A. J. Wing. 1989. "The Incidence of Renal Failure Worldwide and National Statistics for Treatment by Transplantation." In L. Brentand and R. A. Sells, eds., *Organ Transplantation: Current Clinical and Immunological Concepts.* London: Baillire Tindall, 255–69.

Shavelson, L. 1995. *A Chosen Death.* New York: Simon and Schuster.

Shaw, M. W., ed. 1984. *After Barney Clark.* Austin: University of Texas Press.

Sigerist, Henry E. 1943. *Civilization and Disease.* Chicago: University of Chicago Press.

Siminoff, L., A. L. Caplan, R. Arnold, and B. Virnig, B. 1995. "Public Policy Governing Organ and Tissue Procurement." *Annals of Internal Medicine* 123, 1: 10–7.

Singer, P. A. 1975. *Animal Liberation.* New York: Random House.

Singer, P. A. 1992. "Against X Engrafting." *Transplantation Proceedings* 24, 2: 718–22.

Singer, P. A. 1995. *Rethinking Life and Death.* New York: St. Martin's Press.

Singer, P. A., M. Siegler, P. F. Whitington, et al. 1989. "Ethics of Liver Transplantation with Living Donors." *New England Journal of Medicine* 321: 620–22.

Smith, M. D., D. F. Kappell, M. A. Province, et al. 1986. "Living-Related Kidney Donors: A Multicenter Study of Donor Education, Socioeconomic Adjustment and Rehabilitation." *American Journal of Kidney Diseases* 8, 4: 223–33.

Smith, P. 1993. "Family Responsibility and the Nature of Obligation." In D. T. Meyers, K. Kipnis, and C. F. Murphy, Jr., *Kindred Matters.* Ithaca: Cornell University Press, 41–59.

Spece, R. G., D. S. Shimm, and A. E. Buchanan, eds. 1996. *Conflicts of Interest in Clinical Practice and Research.* New York: Oxford University Press.

Specter, M., and G. Kolata. "After Decades and Many Missteps, Cloning Success." 1997. *New York Times,* March 3, A1, B6, 7.

Spital, A. 1991. "The Shortage of Organs for Transplantation: Where Do We Go from Here?" *New England Journal of Medicine* 325, 1243.

Spital, A., and M. Spital. 1985. "Donor's Choice or Hobson's Choice?" *Archives of Internal Medicine* 145: 1297–1301.

Spital, A., and M. Spital. 1988. "Living Kidney Donation." *Archives of Internal Medicine* 148: 1077–80.

Spritz, R., K. Strunk, L. Giebel, and R. King. 1990. "Detection of Mutations in the Tyrosinase Gene in a Patient with Type IA Oculocutaneous Albinism." *New England Journal of Medicine* 322, 24: 1724–28.

Squifflet, J. P., Y. Pirson, A. Poncelet, P. Gianello, and G. Alexandre. 1990. "Unrelated Living Donor Kidney Transplantation." *Transplant International* 3, 1: 32–35.

Starzl, T. E. 1985. "Will Live Organ Donations No Longer Be Justified?" *Hastings Center Report* 15, 2: 5.

Steinbock, B. 1995. "Sperm as Property." *Stanford Law & Policy Review* 57, 2: 57–71.

Stoddard, S. 1978. *The Hospice Movement.* Briarcliff Manor, N.Y.: Stein and Day.

Strong, R. W., S. V. Lynch, T. H. Ong, H. Matsunami, Y. Koido, and G. A. Baldersond. 1990. "Successful Liver Transplantation from a Living Donor to Her Son." *New England Journal of Medicine* 322, 21 (May 24): 1505–1507.

Strunk v. Strunk, 445 S.W. 2d 145 (Ky Ct. App. 1969).

Sun, M. 1988. "EPA Bans Use of Nazi Data." *Science* 240 (September): 20–22.

Swedish Committee on Transplantation. 1989. *Transplantation.* Stockholm: Swedish Ministry of Health and Social Affairs.

Swerdlow, J. L. 1989. *Matching Needs, Saving Lives.* Washington, D.C.: Annenberg.

Szasz, T. 1961. *The Myth of Mental Illness* New York: Harper.

Task Force on Organ Transplantation. 1986. *Organ Transplantation: Issues and Recommendations.* Rockville, Md. Department of Health and Human Services.

Teo, B. 1991. "Organs for Transplantation: The Singapore Experience." *Hastings Center Report* 21, 6: 10–13.

Truog, R. D. 1997. "Is It Time to Abandon Brain Death?" *Hastings Center Report* 27, 1: 29–37.

Truog, R. D., A. S. Brett, and J. Frader. 1992. "The Problem with Futility." *New England Journal of Medicine* 326: 1560–64.

Tufts, A. 1991. "Germany: Calls for Unified Transplantation Law." *Lancet* 337 (June 8): 1403.

Ubel, P., R. Arnold, and A. L. Caplan. 1993. "Rationing Failure: The Ethical Lessons of the Retransplantation of Scarce Vital Organs." *Journal of the American Medical Association* 270 (November 24): 2469–74.

Uniform Anatomical Gift Act *4, 8A ULA 15, 1987.

United States General Accounting Office. 1989. *Heart Transplants: Concerns about Cost, Access and Availability of Donor Organs.* Washington, D.C.: General Accounting Office, HRD 89–61, May.

UNOS Update. 1991. "Alternative Methods to Increasing Organ Donation Presented." 7, 5 (March): 1–5.

Vawter, D. E., K. Gervais, W. Kearney, and A. L. Caplan. 1991. "Fetal Tissue Transplantation and the Problem of Elective Abortion." In W. Land and J. B. Dossetor, eds., *Organ Replacement Therapy.* New York: Springer-Verlag, 491–98.

Vawter, D. E., W. Kearney, K. Gervais, A. L. Caplan, D. Garry, and C. Tauer. 1990. *The Use of Human Fetal Tissue.* Minneapolis: Center for Biomedical Ethics.

Vawter, D. E., and A. L. Caplan. 1992. "Strange Brew: The Ethics and Politics of Fetal Tissue Transplant Research in the United States." *Journal of Laboratory and Clinical Medicine* 120, 1: 30–35.

Veatch, R. M. 1981. "Voluntary Risks to Health: The Ethical Issues." *Journal of the American Medical Association* 243: 50–55.

Veatch, R. M. 1993. "The Impending Collapse of the Whole-Brain Definition of Death." *Hastings Center Report* 23, 4: 18–24.

Wade, N. 1996. "Doctors Question Use of Nazi Medical Atlas." *Canadian Business,* November 26, p. 1.

Walsh, J. 1994. "Reproductive Rights and the Human Genome Project." *Southern California Review of Law and Women's Studies* 145: 160–68.

Walters, L. 1986. "The Ethics of Human Gene Therapy." *Nature* 320 (March 20): 225–27.

Watts, M. 1991. "How People Feel about Organ Donation." Press release, Lieberman, New York.

Weir, R. 1984. *Selective Nontreatment of Handicapped Newborns.* New York: Oxford University Press.

Weir, R., and J. Bale. 1989. "Selective Nontreatment of Neurologically Impaired Neonates." *Neurologic Clinics* 7, 4 (November): 807–20.

Weiss, R. 1997. "Clinton Limits Study of Cloning." *Philadelphia Inquirer,* March 5, A1, 5.

Weiss, S. F. 1987. *Race Hygiene and National Efficiency: The Eugenics of Wilhelm Schallmayer.* Berkeley: University of California Press.

Wertz, D. C., J. H. Fanos, and P. R. Reilly. 1994. "Genetic Testing for Children and Adolescents." *Journal of the American Medical Association* 272, 11: 875–81.

Wight, J. P. 1991. "Ethics, Commerce and Kidneys." *British Medical Journal* 303 (July 13): 110.

Wikler, D. 1988. "The Definition of Death and Persistent Vegetative State." *Hastings Center Report* 18: 44–47.

Wilkie, J. 1991. Personal communication.

Williams, W. 1995. "Boost Organ Donors by Selling Body Parts." *Cincinnati Enquirer,* June 18, p. G3.

Wilmut, I., A. E. Schnieke, J. McWhir, A. J. Kind, and K. H. S. Campbell. 1997. "Viable Offspring Derived from Fetal and Adult Mammalian Cells." *Nature* 385: 810–13.

Witzig, R. 1996. "The Medicalization of 'Race': Scientific Legitimization of a Flawed Social Construct." *Annals of Internal Medicine* 125, 8: 675–79.

Wolstenholme, G., and M. O'Connor, eds. 1968. *Law and Ethics of Transplantation.* London: Ciba Foundation.

Working Group on Mechanical Circulatory Support, National Heart, Lung and Blood Institute. 1985. *Artificial Heart and Assist Devices: Directions, Needs, Costs, Societal and Ethical Issues.* Bethesda, Md.: National Institutes of Health.

World Council of Churches. 1989 *Biotechnology: Its Challenges to the Churches and the World.* Geneva, Switzerland.

World Health Organization. 1991. "Guiding Principles on Human Organ Transplantation." *Lancet* 337 (June 15): 1470–71.

Wozencraft, Ann. 1996. "It's a Baby or It's Your Money Back." *New York Times,* August 25, p. B1.

Wright, R. 1995. "The Trouble with Harry." *New Republic,* July 31, p. 6.

Wyngaarden, J., and L. Smith. 1988. *Cecil Textbook of Medicine.* Philadelphia: Saunders.

Yanaga, K., S. Kakizoe, T. Ikeda, L. G. Podesta, A. Demetris, and T. Starzl. 1990. "Procurement of Liver Allografts from Non-Heart Beating Donors." *Transplantation Proceedings* 22, 1: 275–78.

Young, E., and D. Stevenson. 1990. "Limiting Treatment for Extremely Premature Low Birth Weight Infants." *American Journal of Disabled Children* 144: 549–52.

Youngner, S. 1985. "Psychosocial and Ethical Implications of Organ Retrieval." *New England Journal of Medicine* 313, 5: 321–23.

Youngner, S. J., R. C. Fox, and L. J. O'Connell, eds. 1996. *Organ Transplantation: Meanings and Realities.* Madison: University of Wisconsin Press.

Youngner, S. J., S. Landefeld, C. J. Coulton, et al. 1989. "Brain Death and Organ Retrieval." *Journal of the American Medical Association* 261: 2205–10.

INDEX

Arthur L. Caplan is Trustee Professor of Bioethics and Director, The Center for Bioethics at the University of Pennsylvania. His books include *If I Were a Rich Man, Could I Buy a Pancreas?* (also published by Indiana University Press), *Due Consideration*, and *Moral Matters: Ethical Issues in Medicine and the Life Sciences.* He serves as a member of President Clinton's Presidential Advisory Committee on Gulf War Veterans' Illnesses and as Chair of the Advisory Panel on Blood Safety and Availability for the Department of Health and Human Services/ Food and Drug Administration.